Limb X-ray Interpretation

Limb X-ray Interpretation

Dorthe Larsen RGN, MSc, BSc(HONS), PGCERT(HE)

A&E Department, University Hospital Lewisham

Peter Morris MSc, BSc(HONS)

Bromley Hospitals NHS Trust

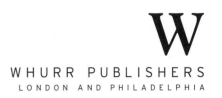

W

WHURR PUBLISHERS
LONDON AND PHILADELPHIA

Copyright © 2006   Whurr Publishers Limited (a subsidiary of John Wiley & Sons Ltd)
                      The Atrium, Southern Gate, Chichester,
                      West Sussex PO19 8SQ, England
                      Telephone   (+44) 1243 779777

Email (for orders and customer service enquiries): cs-books@wiley.co.uk
Visit our Home Page on www.wiley.com

Reprinted October 2006

Designations used by companies to distinguish their products are often claimed as trademarks. All brand
names and product names used in this book are trade names, service marks, trademarks or registered
trademarks of their respective owners. The Publisher is not associated with any product or vendor mentioned in this book.

This publication is designed to provide accurate and authoritative information in regard to the subject
matter covered. It is sold on the understanding that the Publisher is not engaged in rendering professional services. If professional advice or other expert assistance is required, the services of a competent professional should be sought.

Other Wiley Editorial Offices

John Wiley & Sons Inc., 111 River Street, Hoboken, NJ 07030, USA

Jossey-Bass, 989 Market Street, San Francisco, CA 94103-1741, USA

Wiley-VCH Verlag GmbH, Boschstr. 12, D-69469 Weinheim, Germany

John Wiley & Sons Australia Ltd, 42 McDougall Street, Milton, Queensland 4064, Australia

John Wiley & Sons (Asia) Pte Ltd, 2 Clementi Loop #02-01, Jin Xing Distripark, Singapore 129809

John Wiley & Sons Canada Ltd, 22 Worcester Road, Etobicoke, Ontario, Canada M9W 1L1

Wiley also publishes its books in a variety of electronic formats. Some content that appears in print may
not be available in electronic books.

British Library Cataloguing in Publication Data

A catalogue record for this book is available from the British Library

ISBN-13   978-1-86156-499-3 (PB)
ISBN-10   1-86156-499-6 (PB)

Printed and bound in Great Britain by Antony Rowe Ltd, Chippenham, Wiltshire

This book is printed on acid-free paper responsibly manufactured from sustainable forestry in which at
least two trees are planted for each one used for paper production.

Contents

Foreword

It is a pleasure to be able to introduce this new book on injuries to the appendicular skeleton, which combines the basics of clinical assessment with those of plain film interpretation. The book symbolizes the continuing and progressive blurring of boundaries in the provision of patient care; the role of extended-scope practitioners in the evaluation of ambulant patients presenting to emergency departments is of pivotal importance in many departments. It is right that these healthcare professionals should be well informed with regards to the appropriate ordering and interpretation of radiological investigations. The term 'minor injuries' is in some ways a misnomer. The mismanagement of some so-called minor injuries can lead to major morbidity including residual deformity and functional loss for the individual patient – hence the need for high standards of care.

Special features include a lucidly written section on the physics of X-rays and a description of the role of the radiographer in the recognition of radiographic abnormalities. The subsequent chapters follow a format centred around a description of the relevant bony anatomy, the basics of clinical assessment and the clinical features and radiological characteristics of specific injuries.

Dorthe Larsen and Peter Morris have distilled their considerable experience as emergency nurse practitioner and reporting radiographer respectively to produce a book that can be highly recommended not only for the primary target audience of nurse practitioners but also for medical students and junior doctors.

Ashis Banerjee FRCS, FFAEM
Consultant, Emergency Department
University Hospital Lewisham

Preface

Even ten years ago, it was difficult to imagine that this book could have been written, but in the last decade particularly there has been a blurring of previously fixed roles in the hospital team with nurses, radiographers and other professionals allied to medicine taking on roles and responsibilities that were previously the sole domain of doctors. Uniquely, this book is written by a reporting radiographer and a nurse consultant with seven years' experience as an emergency nurse practitioner. The book is intended primarily for any extended-scope practitioners (such as nurse practitioners and physiotherapists) but would also be useful for medical students, junior doctors new to emergency medicine and student reporting radiographers as a reference text in an A&E department or MIU.

Radiographic interpretation is a skill that needs to be acquired, and there is no substitute for experience. However, by following a disciplined and structured approach to analysing a radiograph, most abnormalities can be readily detected and the appropriate treatment given. The aim of this book is to provide practitioners who may have had very little formal radiographic-interpretation training with a guide to appendicular X-ray trauma diagnosis. The content is separated into two distinct parts. Part I addresses technical and professional issues in trauma radiography to help the reader to understand the X-ray process from the initial request for an examination to the final image, including the normal and abnormal appearance of bone on radiographs. In this way, those readers inexperienced in the use of X-rays as a diagnostic tool will gain an appreciation of the responsibilities of the participants involved, and the strengths and limitations of the X-ray examination as a diagnostic tool.

Part II is divided into distinct anatomical regions by chapter. Each chapter follows a similar format with core anatomy linked to the normal radiographic anatomy using radiographs and line diagrams. At times, suggested scan techniques for fracture detection will also be discussed. The common and less common fractures, together with specific radiological signs of abnormalities, mechanism of injury and treatments, are presented with appropriate case studies. Part II concludes with a self-test quiz where the reader can apply the radiographic interpretation techniques suggested.

Dorthe Larsen
Peter Morris

Acknowledgements

This book would never have seen the light of the day without the contributions of several people who deserve our sincere thanks. However, any mistakes or omissions remain firmly our responsibility and should in no way be attributed to them.

We are indebted to all past students that we have had the honour to teach. Your quest for knowledge identified a gap in the literature and provided us with the inspiration to write this book in the first place. We are especially grateful to all the staff and patients who gave permission for their images to be used in this work and to Ashis Banerjee for his helpful comments along the way and for writing the foreword.

Peter would like to thank Dr Drusilla Pearce as clinical director for her support for the project from the outset, Dr Linda Turner and Dr Adrian Thomas for their helpful comments on the manuscript and the reporting radiographers Martha, Mandy, Claire and James for pointing out unusual and interesting films. Dr Adrian Thomas deserves special thanks for providing radiological mentorship to the reporting radiographer service without which this role extension simply would not have happened.

Finally, to my wife, Lucy, and our children – thank you for all your love and support.

Dorthe would like to thank Yvonne Burns (ENP) for her generosity in sharing her vast knowledge and experience, especially in the early stages, Debra Illott for her 'red pen', critical eye and wit, and her work colleagues (especially Carole Ambrose, Carol Spanswick, Sarah Carver and the ENP team) for accepting her one and only excuse when priorities changed and for giving so much support and encouragement. Special thanks must go to Rob Forman for saving the hard drive when the computer crashed and we had no back-up copy!

Finally, to my friends, family and especially Shaun Swaby – thank you for your love, support and for allowing me to give up the time I should have spent with you to work on this book.

Part I

Technical and Professional Issues

Chapter 1
The basic principles of radiology

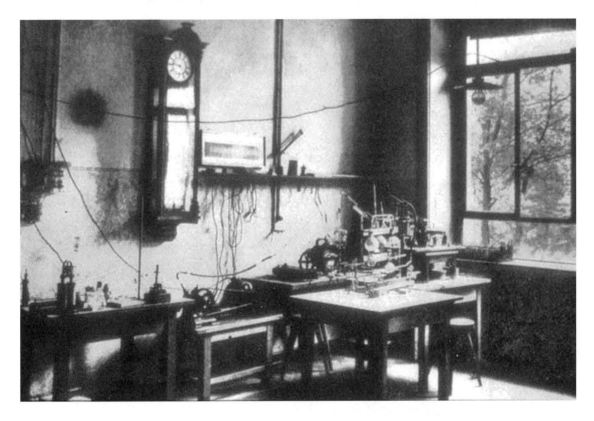

Figure 1.1 Physical Institute laboratory at Würzburg in which Röntgen first noted and investigated X-rays. (Reproduced with kind permission, (c) Radiology Centennial Inc.)

We are all probably aware that we are surrounded every moment of every day by different forms of radiation. In fact, the world is constantly bombarded by cosmic radiation of varying wavelengths. Light, of course, is the most obvious and readily appreciated form; but in November 1895 Professor Wilhelm Röntgen of the University of Würzburg discovered a type of radiation that had been previously unknown to science. He noticed that some apparatus he was experimenting with caused chemically impregnated cardboard to glow, even though the equipment itself was completely covered in black card;

furthermore, when his hand was between the equipment and the cardboard, he could see a likeness of the bones projected as a shadow within the outline of his hand. He soon discovered that the effect occurred through a thick book, wooden planks and even metal sheets. Röntgen named the cause of this phenomenon 'X-rays', on the basis that he did not know what was the actual cause, and this name has continued to the present day. He had discovered a type of radiation with the property of selective absorption: certain materials, such as metal and bone, absorb more X-rays than others, such as air, water and organic soft tissues, which instead allow more of the X-ray beam to pass unabsorbed. In this way, the bones of his hand appeared to be denser than the other, non-mineralized, soft tissues, such as muscle, tendon and cartilage. Thus, one of the most significant and far-reaching advances in science in recent decades came about fortuitously. Over the next few years, he explored the physics associated with his discovery and, in particular, developed medical applications. In 1901, Röntgen was awarded the Nobel Prize for physics.

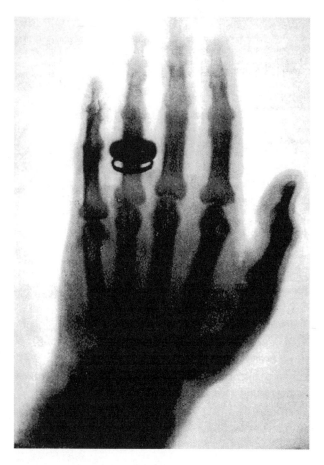

Figure 1.2 Often incorrectly described as the first ever radiograph, this is allegedly Mrs Röntgen's hand taken on 22 December 1895. (Reproduced with kind permission, (c) Radiology Centennial Inc.)

It did not take long for the medical establishment to recognize the value of rendering deeper anatomical structures visible, and many hospitals acquired X-ray apparatus shortly after the initial discovery. However, because of the low power of the apparatus, exposure times were very long; in 1896, a chest X-ray of a 10-year-old girl was taken at London's St Thomas's hospital with an exposure time of 30 minutes. What were not initially appreciated were the harmful effects of X-rays on human tissue. Many of the early pioneers of the techniques developed signs of skin damage and had hands or arms amputated; some subsequently died of radiation-induced disease. There was, of course, no inkling of radiation protection; indeed, it was common practice for X-ray operators to test the apparatus with their own hands (Thomas, 1995).

Some of the limitations of this 'plain' X-ray technique were soon overcome by the administration of contrast media, i.e. substances which are relatively opaque to X-rays and which would reveal specifically targeted soft tissues. From these early experiments – some of which were fatal – many of the examinations that are commonplace today were developed. For example, rectal administration of barium sulphate gives excellent visualization of the lining of the large bowel and is superb in the diagnosis of colonic cancers; this examination is known now, of course, as the barium enema.

Nowadays, exactly the same properties and principles are employed by modern medical X-ray departments to provide a range of imaging *modalities* and techniques that are used to investigate disease and pathology. In turn, other, non-X-ray-based modalities have since been developed, such as Ultrasound and Magnetic Resonance Imaging (MRI), to the extent that we now have departments of 'Imaging' rather than simply 'X-ray'. Examinations have become interventional as well as simply diagnostic; disease can now be treated under X-ray guidance to, e.g. open diseased arteries, remove kidney or gall stones, embolize (stop) internal bleeding, extract samples of tissue from deep structures for biopsy and almost countless other techniques. However, the plain film X-ray investigation is still very often the first referral for an imaging examination and is the frontline investigative tool in A&E departments and MIUs for cases of trauma. There is also the major field of tumour treatment using high-power X-ray machines, a technique known as radiotherapy. In addition, radiography is now also used for many diverse industrial purposes, such as airport security, metal-welding integrity and for the investigation of art and museum artefacts. In order to fully appreciate the strengths and weaknesses of the X-ray image (hereafter referred to as a *radiograph*) as such a tool, a basic understanding of the process of generating a radiograph is necessary. It is not the purpose of this chapter to make medical physicists of us all but merely to give a practical grasp of the essential principles of image production and of the factors which degrade that image.

The production of radiographs

The production of a radiograph, although an apparently quick and accessible medical examination, is actually rather costly and relies on some extremely complex, dedicated equipment. A modern radiology department is easily the most expensive department to equip and maintain in any hospital. The basic principle is, however, reasonably straightforward. Firing an electron beam at a tungsten target generates an X-ray beam. The electrons interact with the tungsten and a product of a single interaction is the emission of an X-ray *photon*. The electrical energy originally possessed by the electron is therefore converted into X-ray energy. By careful construction of the X-ray-generating device (generally known as the *X-ray* tube as it is contained within a glass envelope or tube from which the air has been removed – see Figure 1.3 below), a beam of X-rays can be made to emerge from a port in the tube and be directed towards the object of interest. Lead shielding absorbs X-rays that emerge in an unwanted direction. When the beam is directed towards an object, there will be absorption of a proportion of the beam by the object.

This absorption of X-ray photons from the beam is known as *attenuation*. If the object is uniform, such as a sheet of metal or paper, there will be a uniform attenuation of X-rays emerging from the object. The

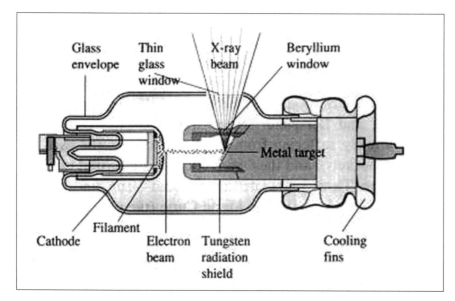

Figure 1.3 Schematic diagram of typical X-ray tube. Note the electron beam strikes the tungsten target and is converted into a beam of X-ray photons.

amount of attenuation will depend directly on the properties and thickness of the material being penetrated. If a sheet of photographic film is placed in the path of the emerging beam, a blackening of the film will occur. Therefore, if an object is more complex than a uniform sheet and is composed of materials of different absorptive properties, a shadow of this object will be cast on the photographic film, with more blackening occurring in those areas of film where the greater amount of X-rays have fallen. Figure 1.3 (above) shows a schematic representation of an X-ray tube and emerging beam. This, then, is the basic principle of the production of a radiograph: a beam of X-rays is directed towards an object, some of the X-ray beam is absorbed by the object and that which is not completely absorbed is used to blacken sensitive photographic film and produce an image of the object.

The X-ray tube and associated components are contained within a manoeuvrable housing, which is either floor- or, more commonly now, ceiling-mounted in a specially constructed X-ray room. This allows the radiographer to direct the X-ray beam towards the affected anatomical region of the patient. Bear in mind that the patient may present as a walking, co-operative individual or as an incapacitated trolley patient. The tube housing must therefore be able to be positioned at all sorts of angles, heights and directions in order to achieve a successful radiograph, and this relies on substantial and complex engineering for the required manoeuvrability. The electrical generating equipment required is itself substantial as the voltages and power required are considerable. The voltage generators are housed in large cabinets in the X-ray room, which will have a dedicated electrical supply to cope with the high power consumption. At the time of writing this chapter, the installation of a modern general X-ray room will cost upwards of £300,000. Additionally, the equipment itself is so heavy that the floors and ceilings of X-ray rooms have to be specially strengthened, again adding to the overall cost to the hospital for this facility.

The production of a useful image

Probably everyone who has either 'had an X-ray' or who has seen one is aware that radiographs are most commonly used to examine bones. But why are X-rays especially useful for imaging the bony skeleton? And why are they generally less useful for looking at the soft tissues?

The absorption of X-rays by any given material depends on two main factors: the atomic number of the constituent atoms and the density of the substance. The atomic number, without straying too far into a discussion of quantum physics, is a measure of the number of components of an atom of the substance concerned. Lead has an atomic number of 82, whereas carbon has an atomic number of 6. When an X-ray photon interacts with the atoms in a substance, it is either absorbed completely or deflected ('scattered') from its original path. If it does not interact at all, in other words the photon misses all the atoms in the thickness of material through which it is directed, there will be no attenuation of the X-ray beam due to this process. Materials with very high atomic numbers, such as metals and in particular lead, absorb almost all the X-rays, and there will be a high degree of beam attenuation. This is because there is a very high chance of an interaction occurring rather than not occurring; similarly, the greater the density of the material, the greater the degree of beam attenuation. Conversely, the lower the atomic number, the less dense the material is, or the thinner the material, the less chance there is of our hypothetical X-ray photon interacting with the material. Therefore, more of the beam passes through the material, and the attenuation of the beam is low. Typical examples of materials causing low beam attenuation are water, air or wood. Of particular significance to medical radiology are two facts:

1. The atomic number of bone is twice that of soft tissues (14 as against 7.5)
2. The density of bone is 1.8 times that of soft tissues

With the power levels used for diagnostic medical X-rays, the difference of the atomic numbers has a particularly profound effect and results in bone very significantly attenuating the X-ray beam compared with soft tissues. Figure 1.4 (below) schematically illustrates this point.

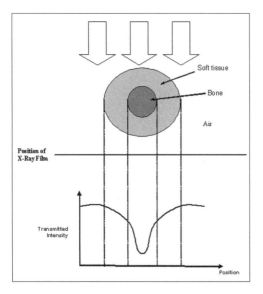

Figure 1.4 Schematic diagram of a uniform X-ray beam interacting with a section of limb consisting of soft tissue and bone. The graph below shows the transmitted intensity of the beam emerging from the limb. That part of the beam which interacts only with air is at the highest intensity. Those parts that pass through the tissue are attenuated: the amount of attenuation depends on the thickness as well as the type of tissue; the part that passes through the middle of the bone will have the least intensity when emerging from the patient.

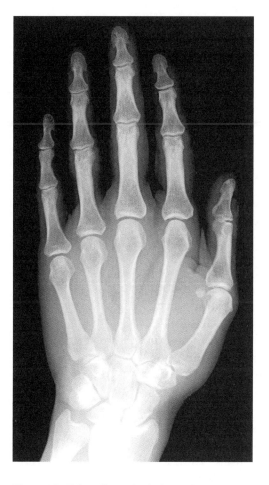

Figure 1.5 This radiograph of a hand demonstrates the grey-scale range for tissues, from almost black representing air to the dense cortical bone shown as white. The soft tissues are represented by intermediate greys.

When a uniform X-ray beam moves towards a complex object such as a human limb, the emerging beam is no longer uniform. It is now made up of areas of different amounts of X-ray photons, and these photons will have a range of energies. What exists, in fact, is a *latent image* of the structures through which the X-ray beam has passed. When this is rendered visible by use of some sort of X-ray-sensitive recording medium, such as photographic film, the useful information from the radiograph can be gleaned.

In order that the visible image is of diagnostic quality, the intensity of the beam which actually forms the image on the X-ray film must be within certain limits, depending on the properties of the film. If the intensity of the beam is too great, too much blackening of the film occurs and the image is said to be *over-exposed*. Even the densest anatomical structures will have been over-penetrated and detail of the object will have been lost. Conversely, if the intensity of the beam is too low, too little blackening will occur and, again, detail of the anatomical structures will be inadequate and the film is said to be *under-exposed*. The beam intensity is varied by adjusting certain exposure factors at the X-ray tube control panel; these are set by the radiographer at the time of the exposure and will depend on the anatomical region under examination and the age and physical size of the patient. These factors include the energy imparted to the X-ray photon, the number of photons for a given time and the overall time of the exposure. The selection of exposure factors is something of an art, learned by the radiographer through practice and experience, since radiography is essentially a blind technique (in other words, the results are only seen once the image is processed and an incorrect choice of exposure factors will therefore necessitate a repeat examination).

In summary, when an anatomical structure is examined using X-rays, an image is produced with the densest structures, normally bone, conventionally showing as white and the least-dense structures such as thin soft tissue regions or particularly air-filled structures showing as black. Of course, even a human limb consists of structures comprising a range of densities, and there will similarly be a range of blackening on a radiograph from black right across the grey-scale to white for the densest bone.

Radiographic recording media

Conventional film

The very earliest radiographs were viewed on fluorescent screens and, necessarily, in almost complete darkness. This was due to the low power of the equipment available and the insensitivity of the photographic films of the time. However, by the early twentieth century, images were viewed as photographic negatives on, initially, glass plates and later on flexible film. Until very recently this was the only way to view and store radiographic images. The emerging X-ray beam, having passed through an object and therefore comprising a latent image, is directed towards photographic film; the X-ray photons interact with the film emulsion and, when chemically processed in much the same way as conventional photographic film, a visible and permanent image appears that can then be stored for as long as necessary. We are all familiar with these films that are viewed on a light box – a viewer containing fluorescent tubes which provide an even spread of white light to illuminate the film.

As radiographic techniques developed and improved, images of very high quality became possible, the causes of un-sharpness were minimized and exposure times shortened from the very earliest of, not unusually, several hours to the present times of a few thousandths of a second. The film used is housed in a lightproof cassette that nowadays also includes intensifying screens to maximize the conversion of the X-ray beam into a visible image on the film. Processing the image has also developed; long gone are the days of a darkroom with a technician who processed images in tanks of developer, rinse and fixer. With current technology, processors exist that can take the cassette, posted by the radiographer into the front of the machine, open it, remove, process and dry the film and return the cassette loaded with a fresh film, all within 45 seconds.

Computerized radiography

Inevitably, computers and microprocessors have become inextricably embedded in the acquisition of radiographic images. Probably the single greatest development since the initial discovery of X-rays is the

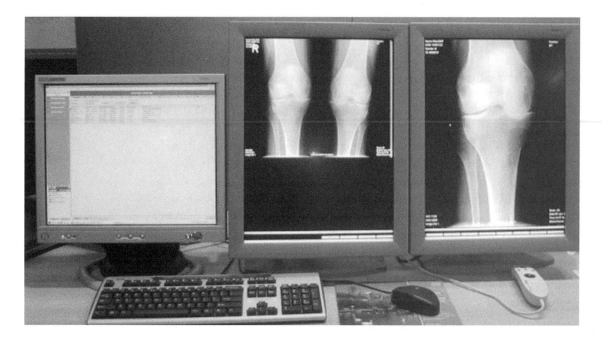

Figure 1.6 Computer workstation used to view radiographs on the PACS network. (Reproduced with kind permission, Rogan-Delft BV, Holland)

Computed Radiography System and PACS. Instead of a cassette containing photographic film, the recording media is an imaging plate that is capable of being read by a computer. The image produced is sent to a workstation for manipulation by the radiographer, who can adjust brightness and contrast, annotate with text, crop or enlarge and make other adjustments to the final image. This is then sent on to the hospital network for viewing on workstations around the hospital or even remotely at other sites by the clinicians. This has revolutionized the working practice in the hospitals that have adopted these systems; X-ray departments need no longer provide large film stores to hold the millions of images stored in cardboard film packets. Transportation of the heavy film packets is eliminated. Practitioners in different parts of the hospital or even in different hospitals can view images simultaneously. Theoretically, the likelihood of an image being lost is greatly reduced (no more film packets hiding in the boot of a consultant's car). There is also much greater latitude in the required exposure: the computer can compensate for a certain amount of over- or under-exposure thereby lessening the guestimate of exposure factors by the radiographer. Interestingly, though, computerized radiography does not eliminate the image artefacts that are demonstrable in conventional film. In fact, there are image aberrations that *only* appear in CR.

Radiographic appearance of different materials, shapes and forms

As has been mentioned above, the degree of attenuation of an X-ray beam passing through an object depends on several properties of the object material. But how does this translate to the actual appearance on the resultant radiograph? A crucial point to remember is that a radiograph is a two-dimensional representation of a three-dimensional object. Look at the radiograph of a chicken's egg in Figure 1.7. It is essentially uniform, apart from the blacker region at the right. An unfertilized egg is completely filled with fluid, except at one end where there is an air sac. This is represented by the blacker area; air is less dense than the fluid, thus more X-rays penetrate this region and therefore give a greater blackening of the film. Notice also that the fluid bulges into the air sac, giving a crescent of composite shadowing where the X-ray beam passes through air first, then fluid and then air again, resulting in an intermediate image density.

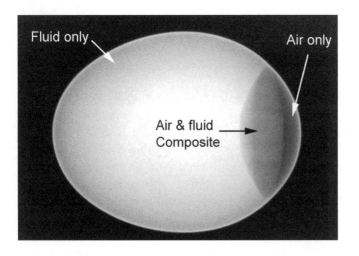

Figure 1.7 Radiograph of a chicken's egg showing different image densities where the beam has passed through fluid only, air only or a region of composite air and fluid resulting in an intermediate image density. Note also the fine increase in density at the periphery as the X-ray beam passes through the shell of the egg tangentially.

Not quite so obvious, perhaps, is the thin, dense (white) rim of the egg. This is because the thin shell is curving away from the X-ray beam's source and the beam is passing tangentially through the shell. The shell includes calcium salts, which are relatively opaque to X-rays and thus the circumference of the egg is actually the most *radiopaque* and therefore appears most dense on the resultant radiograph. This is directly analogous to the radiographic appearance of the cortex of a long bone. This also shows densest at the margin of the bone where the X-ray beam has passed tangentially through the compact cortical bone. Remember also that the egg is a three-dimensional object – egg-shaped – whose centre is fattest and provides a greater thickness of material through which the beam must pass. That is why the egg is not completely uniform in density but appears white at the centre and greyer towards the periphery.

Look at the radiographs of a light bulb in Figure 1.8. Although they appear similar, the image on the left has been made with X-rays of a higher penetrating power. Notice how detail at the base of the light bulb is much clearer, owing to the greater penetration of the metal by the higher-power X-ray beam. Note also the glass bulb is only clearly shown at its periphery where the X-ray beam passes through the glass tangentially and therefore at much greater relative thickness than the centre. This shows more clearly than the eggshell seen in Figure 1.7 because the light bulb contains a partial vacuum rather than fluid, as in the egg. The light bulb was X-rayed in its cardboard box, which is again only demonstrated along the edges.

X-rays are often requested to search for penetrating foreign bodies (see Figure 1.9). Although they can be invaluable for locating foreign bodies containing certain materials that are dense enough to be demonstrated on radiographs, many simply are not shown. In particular, wood and most plastics are of similar density to soft tissues and will not be visible on the image and therefore there is insufficient image *contrast* to render the object visible.

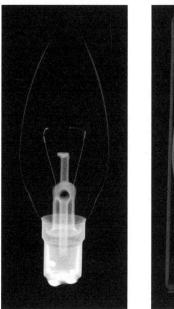
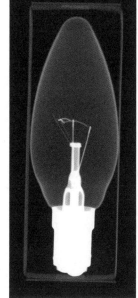

Figure 1.8 Two radiographs of a light bulb using different exposure factors. The image on the left was taken with a beam of higher penetrating power and hence has revealed detail not evident in the image on the right.

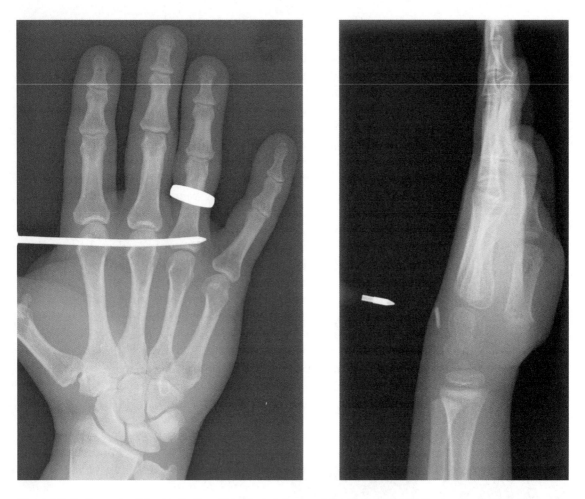

Figure 1.9 Radiographs of foreign bodies within the soft tissues of the hand. Note how the greater density of the metal nail on the left prevents a blackening of the film and results in a very white image, whereas the less-dense glass sliver on the right image appears grey.

When requesting X-rays for penetrating or locating ingested foreign bodies, it is useful to be able to know how the foreign body might appear. For example, certain ingested fish bones (cod or mackerel) will show in the throat because of the calcific content of the bone, whereas others, such as dogfish (rock salmon), are composed of cartilage with no ossification and will be invisible. All the examples of foreign-body materials so far mentioned give positive contrast on the image, i.e. they are denser than the surrounding tissues. Air and fat both result in negative contrast and appear blacker on the image. A penetrating injury will often show air within the soft tissues, and fat leaking from a fractured long bone will also show blacker than blood (see lipohaemarthrosis in the knee – Chapter 8).

Summary

- Radiographs are produced by firing a beam of electrons within an X-ray tube at a tungsten target. The result is a beam of X-rays that can be directed at a region of the body.
- The image is produced by a process of selective absorption whereby denser structures such as skeletal bones absorb more X-rays, attenuating the beam and creating whiter areas on the image than the less-dense structures (which appear grey or even black).
- The degree of beam attenuation and therefore image density depends on the atomic number and density of the target material as well as the shape, size and thickness of the structure.
- The radiographer controls the penetrating power and amount of X-rays within the beam – the exposure factors – to suit the part of the body under examination. The selection of correct exposure factors is crucial when producing a diagnostic image.
- Radiographs can be recorded on transparent photographic film or on a computer-read imaging plate, which allows the image to be viewed via the hospital's computer network.
- X-ray examinations can be used to demonstrate a foreign body, but only certain materials that are of sufficiently different density to the soft tissues will show on the resultant image.

Suggested further reading

For a concise and very readable history of the discovery and development of X-rays and radiology see *The Invisible Light: 100 Years of Medical Radiology*, edited by Adrian Thomas (Blackwell Science, 1995). For those interested in X-ray physics, Robin Wilks's *The Principles of Radiological Physics* (Churchill Livingstone, 1994) gives a good in-depth account. *Squire's Fundamentals of Radiology* by Robert A Novelline (Harvard University Press, 1997) has some nice images that further demonstrate the principles of image contrast, shape and form.

Chapter 2

Professional issues in radiography

X-ray requesting

This is the start of the process in generating a medical radiograph for diagnostic purposes. The original X-ray requests were effectively a question from one doctor to another concerning a patient; the clinician, having examined the patient, asks the radiologist for an expert opinion. Nowadays, the referral (request) for a radiological opinion is not restricted only to doctors, but is regulated by the Ionising Radiation (Medical Exposure) Regulation Act of 2000, where the referrer is defined as: 'a registered medical practitioner, dental practitioner or other health care professionals who is entitled in accordance with the employer's procedure, to refer individuals for medical exposure to a practitioner' (Department of Health and Royal College of Nursing, 2003: 36) – in this case, a radiographer or radiologist. It is now commonplace for nurses, physiotherapists and other health care professionals to request a radiological opinion, and access to diagnostic tests has also been highlighted as one of the ten key roles for both nurses (Department of Health, 2000) and, more recently, allied health professionals (Department of Health, 2003).

One of the key roles of the radiographer is to validate the request, ensuring that sufficient information is given by the referrer to justify the exposure to the patient (Bowman and Sloane, 1999). The referrer must obtain an in-depth history, including mechanism of injury together with a thorough clinical examination, to satisfy the above regulation and prevent any inappropriate investigations being carried out. Swelling is often gravitational and may not represent the actual site of the injury. Imagine a patient with an upper-limb fracture where the arm has not been elevated. The hand will be swollen and simply to X-ray it will inevitably lead to a missed fracture. It is good practice to adopt the standard orthopaedic examination principle of the 'joint above and joint below' the site of the patient's complaint so as to reduce the risk of missing any injuries. Some injuries occur in recognized patterns, e.g. a fracture to the ulna with dislocation of the radial head. Finally, X-rays should only ever be undertaken for clinical correlation, where the result will positively or negatively affect the management plan. The management plan for a patient with a clinically fractured rib (without any lung involvement) remains the same regardless of radiological findings, thus rendering an X-ray unnecessary.

Many A&E departments have introduced nurse-led X-ray requesting at triage, which has proven to reduce the patient's overall journey time (Lindsey-Jones and Finlayson, 2000) and high levels of staff and patient satisfaction (Chudleigh, 2004). This initiative is also supported by the *Reforming Emergency Care* (Department of Health, 2001) document which ensures that patients are seen, treated, discharged or admitted within the required four hours. The literature reveals that nurses can do this effectively with appropriate training (Chudleigh, 2004), although in some places the requesting protocols can be limited to certain anatomical areas (such as wrist and ankle) excluding others (such as elbow and knee) with no good clinical justification. This can potentially lead to associated injuries being missed or the patient being returned to X-ray at a later stage, thus negating the initiative.

Several studies have demonstrated nurse practitioners' ability to request and interpret radiographs correctly (Allerston and Justham, 2000; Overton-Brown and Anthony, 1998; Meek et al., 1998), and yet these nurse practitioners are being hindered in doing so in many hospitals. One study highlighted that while 84% of nurse practitioners in the UK could request X-rays only 36% were allowed to interpret them (Tye et al., 1998). Dolan (2000) describes this as patients being used as pawns in a game of professional chess. Under the current Government, the NHS went through yet another organizational change, which this time also included a redesign of the workforce (Davies, 2003). The aim of this redesign is to create a more patient-centred health care system and to do away with the historically closely guarded demarcation of professional roles (Lissauer, 2003). Sir George Alberti (National Director for Emergency Access, Department of Health) argues that many of the obstacles facing NHS staff are based on myths and a failure to interpret professional guidance rather than legal restriction (Department of Health and Royal College of Nursing, 2003). Evidence of reformed working practices are emerging, with many well-publicised innovative nurse-led services (Department of Health and Royal College of Nursing, 2003), but less-well-publicised advanced roles in radiography. The most common myth in radiology must be that only doctors can request an X-ray, which we have already dispelled, or that radiographers only 'take the picture'/run the scanner. The reality is that many places have radiographers engaged in a wide range of advanced activities, such as performing and reporting on barium enemas, flexible sigmoidoscopy with biopsy and poplypectomy as required and reporting ultra-sonography (Cameron and Masterson, 2003; Snaith et al., 2004).

The 'red dot' system

Currently, it is common for hospitals to operate the 'red dot' system for examining radiographers to indicate to A&E staff that they suspect an abnormality has been demonstrated on an examination. In practical terms, this means that if a radiographer is suspicious of a fracture or other pathology a red dot is placed on the film or the film packet. This useful system was first used in 1981, when senior radiographers at the Ealing Hospital instigated the practice of marking film packets with a red dot. The intention was to draw on the practical experience of the examining radiographer in order to contribute to a good outcome for the patient by hopefully reducing the number of missed abnormalities. The scheme was set up with careful consideration and discussion and included the following four points clearly stated in a letter (Cheyne et al., 1987) to the A&E department from the senior consultant radiologist:

1. This is not the diagnosis of an abnormality and has no legal or professional importance: it merely states that the radiographer concerned suspects that there may be an abnormality on the film.
2. The absence of such a mark does not imply that the radiographer considers that there is no suspicion of abnormality on the film.
3. The responsibility for examining the film, in the first instance, and deciding on the management of the patient rests and continues to rest with the referrer concerned.
4. The system is meant to represent no more than a helpful informal signal to the referrer on the basis of the radiographic and practical experience of the radiographers concerned.

Although the roles of A&E and radiographic staff have moved on since then, e.g. casualty officers are not the only staff now to refer for X-ray, these sentiments are certainly as valid today as in 1981, and should be borne in mind by the referrer when viewing films so marked. We believe that the red dot system is a very sensible use of the experience of the radiographer; however, it must be used as it was always meant to be used: as an informal assistance rather than as an absolute indication of the presence or otherwise of disease. Currently, some hospitals have an extension of this system whereby the radiographer makes a written comment rather than simply red-dotting the film. It must be remembered that this is not a formal report. The experience of the radiographer, as with any other hospital staff, will vary greatly between individuals; workload also plays a part – if the radiographer is working single-handed and is very busy, there may not be time to scour every examination for an abnormality as if they were providing a formal report.

Figure 2.1 AP shoulder view that was originally marked with a red dot in order to indicate a suspected abnormality – see text for explanation.

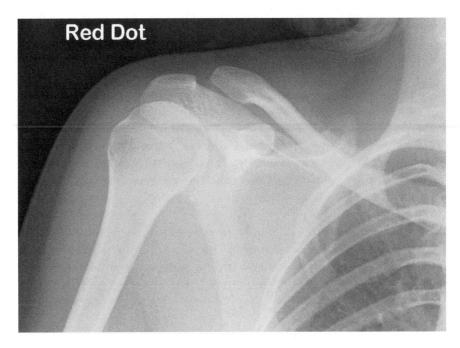

As an example of the potential for failure of the red dot, consider the radiograph in Figure 2.1. This patient was a teenage girl who had fallen from her horse. The radiographer marked this film with a red dot because of a misalignment of the acromio-clavicular joint indicating subluxation. Unfortunately, the film was initially interpreted as representing a posterior gleno-humeral dislocation, after all the humeral head does appear somewhat symmetrical – the classic 'light bulb' sign. However, the second (axial) view which was available at the time absolutely confirmed that there was no dislocation. The misdiagnosis would have been avoided had, first, the reason for the red dot been ascertained with the examining radiographer and, second, had the axial view been checked.

The radiological report

In 1995, the Royal College of Radiologists made a recommendation that every radiographic examination should be accompanied by a written report that is timely, accurate and appropriate. In an A&E/MIU setting, the X-ray examination is carried out and the resulting radiographs inspected by the clinician followed by treatment or management based on the findings of the examination together with information from the clinical examination and other diagnostic tests.

After the patient has been treated and/or discharged, the radiographs are then returned to the X-ray department where they are collated and reported. Traditionally, this second look was done by a radiologist and resulted in a written expert opinion on the presence or otherwise of pathology on the radiographs. Copies of this report are kept with the X-ray film packet – or electronic equivalent – and also in the patient's notes or casualty attendance card. Any discrepancies – i.e. missed fractures or pathologies – can then be addressed and the patient recalled as necessary. This report is a professional expert opinion of what the radiographic image shows. Currently, however, many X-ray departments are unable to provide the radiological support to report all plain films in as timely a fashion as would be desirable. The reasons for this difficulty are varied: the demands on radiologists' time are huge with departments becoming ever busier, the examinations performed in X-ray departments are many and diverse with newer modalities such as CT and MRI generating complex images taking priority, more interventional work, fewer consultant radiologists being appointed and so on.

In order to address this issue, many hospitals have extended the roles of radiographers to include some of the more routine radiological workload, such as plain X-ray reporting and ultrasound. Reporting radiographers, after completion of a postgraduate course in skeletal radiographic interpretation, report plain radiographs requested by A&E or GPs. This report may be written either at the time the image was obtained ('hot reporting') or when the image is returned to the radiology department ('cold reporting'), a role previously only undertaken by radiologists (Bowman and Sloane, 1999). At Pinderfields General Hospital, specially trained radiographers 'hot report' all plain film radiographs from A&E (Snaith et al., 2004). As only 25% of all A&E departments' attendances will have a radiological abnormality, patients at Pinderfields are referred from A&E to X-ray by a clinician (doctor or nurse practitioner) with a management plan. If no abnormalities are found, the radiographer will discharge the patient in accordance with the management plan (Snaith et al., 2004). During the first ten weeks of this service, 914 'hot reports' were made with 58% discharges by radiographers, leading to a significant reduction in the patient's overall journey time in A&E and the increased clinical decision-making process by the radiographer. It is crucial to understand that the report written by a radiographer is not inferior to that written by a radiologist; the quality of the reports should be indistinguishable. However, the radiographer does not have the same extensive medical training, experience and knowledge as the radiologist and will therefore not report on all films. For example, those films showing a malignant pathological process should be shown to a radiologist, who is better placed to comment on the significance of the appearances and make the necessary appropriate referrals.

There will normally be a scheme of work in place agreed by the departmental clinical director and the relevant trust authority to allow radiographers to report. This scheme details the types of films – appendicular, axial, chest etc. – and also the referral source such as A&E or general practice that the radiographers may report to.

Radiation protection

The early radiology pioneers had no inkling of the detrimental effect of the exposure of human tissue to uncontrolled doses of X-ray radiation. In fact, it was common practice for the operator to test the X-ray beam using his or her own hands. There was even a technique of 'hardening' the beam by using the operator's own hand as a filter to remove the softer (lower power) X-rays and thereby improve the quality of the final image. It was soon realized, however, that the X-rays were not completely benign, as was first thought, when the radiological pioneers started to exhibit unpleasant symptoms (see Figure 2.2, below).

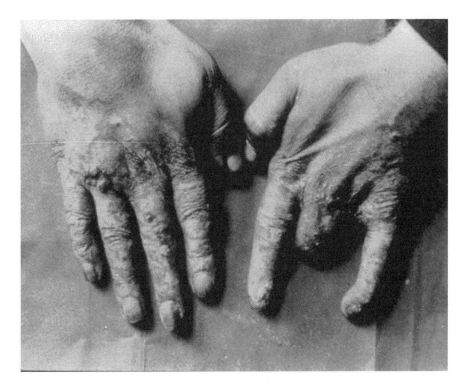

Figure 2.2 The hands of Mihran Kassabian (1870–1910), an early radiology pioneer who photographed the progressive necrozing effects of unprotected exposure to radiation on his own tissues. (Reproduced with kind permission, © Radiology Centennial Inc.)

We know that the interaction of X-ray photons with tissue causes damage and this damage occurs at the molecular level, the cellular level and at organ level. Exposure to the low levels of radiation typical to medical radiography does not cause radiation burns or radiation sickness. The only known effect is a slight increase in the chance of a cancer occurring later in life. It is impossible to give an absolute prediction that given a certain X-ray dose a cancer will occur. It is therefore usual to calculate the likely statistical increase in the chance of a patient developing a cancer over and above that chance which everybody has, which is approximately one in three over a normal lifetime. In other words, what is the *possible* extra chance of developing a cancer at some stage as in addition to the one in three? Figure 2.3 shows the relative risks of some typical medical X-ray examinations. Note that each examination is given a comparison with the natural background radiation to which we are all exposed.

The technological progress in X-ray equipment and recording media over the years has permitted a huge reduction in the radiation dose for medical examinations without any loss of technical performance. Over the last thirty years or so, there has been a further drive to reduce unnecessary radiation exposure by applying a risk/benefit strategy to X-ray requesting. In other words, if the X-ray examination is not going to benefit the patient by providing useful information, the examination should not be performed. The Ionising Radiation (Medical Exposure) Regulation 2000 (known colloquially as 'Irmer') is the statutory instrument regulating the use of ionizing radiation for medical purposes. In particular, it defines the roles of those staff in the examination process. Briefly these roles are as follows:

Referrer

The referrer is a 'registered medical practitioner, dental practitioner or other health professional who is entitled in accordance with the employer's procedures to refer individuals for medical exposure to a practitioner'. This is the person making the request for an X-ray examination.

Practitioner

This is usually a consultant radiologist who authorizes the request for an X-ray and is able to justify that it is of benefit to the patient on the basis of the information included in the request. Although the legal responsibility remains with the radiologist, in practice the radiographer takes on the role of practitioner and authorizes the exposure when plain X-ray examinations are requested.

Operator

This is the person physically operating the equipment concerned. It is the duty of the operator to identify the patient correctly, ensure that the procedure has been justified by a practitioner, check for pregnancy

X-ray examination (Nuclear medicine or isotope scan)	Equivalent period of natural background radiation	Lifetime additional risk of cancer per examination*
Chest Teeth Arms and legs Hands and feet	A few days	NEGLIGIBLE RISK Less than 1 in 1,000,000
Skull Head Neck	A few weeks	MINIMAL RISK 1 in 1,000,000 to 1 in 100,000
Breast [mammography] Hip Spine Abdomen Pelvis CT scan of head (Lung isotope scan) (Kidney isotope scan)	A few months to a year	VERY LOW RISK 1 in 100,000 to 1 in 10,000
Kidneys and bladder [IVU] Stomach – barium meal Colon – barium enema CT scan of chest CT scan of abdomen (Bone isotope scan)	A few years	LOW RISK 1 in 10,000 to 1 in 1,000

Figure 2.3 Relative radiation dose and risks for diagnostic X-ray examinations. (Reproduced with kind permission, National Radiological Protection Board)

* These risk levels represent very small additions to the 1 in 3 chance we all have of getting cancer

status etc. The practitioner and the operator may be the same person.

In day-to-day practice in the X-ray department, there are many ways to minimize X-ray doses to patients. The most, perhaps glaringly, obvious way is to ensure that the patient hasn't already been examined for the same complaint. There is no sense in obtaining an additional radiograph if no further injury has taken place. If the examination took place in a different hospital, the effort should be made to obtain copies or a formal report. Avoid, particularly in children, examining the opposite limb for comparison. It is better to get an experienced opinion, e.g. from a radiologist or senior A&E doctor, first. Try and avoid multiple requests; e.g. 'hand, wrist and elbow' or 'ankle and foot'. Clinical examination should identify the specific area of interest; it is rare to see separate fractures in both ankle and foot – remember the base of the fifth metatarsal should always be demonstrated on the lateral ankle view.

The X-ray room installation and equipment is designed to minimize unnecessary exposure to patients and staff. The radiographer will use good practice to minimize dose, e.g. collimating (restricting) the X-ray beam to the area of interest and within the cassette, using lead protective sheets over radiosensitive tissues where appropriate, making the correct selection of exposure factors, ensuring a good positioning and appropriate projections to avoid repeats. In essence, if the principle of a radiation dose – 'as low as reasonably achievable' (ALARA) – is adopted, the risk/benefit ratio will be favourable.

Further useful information is available at the website of the National Radiological Protection Board at www.nrpb.org.

Chapter 3

The normal and abnormal appearance of bone on radiographs

Bone is a dynamic, living tissue that performs several functions. It gives form and shape to a living structure, provides mechanical strength and protection; provides attachment points for the anchoring of muscles and other soft tissues and, by articulating with other bones at various joints, allows a wide range of movement. Additionally, it provides a reservoir of specific minerals, principally calcium and phosphorus. Fat cells are stored within the bone, providing a source of energy; and bone marrow in certain bones produces blood cells and platelets. It grows as the individual matures and is capable of repair following injury. This chapter is concerned with the appearance of normal and abnormal or diseased bone on radiographs and the description and classification of these appearances. It is not a comprehensive analysis or description of bone physiology, and the reader is advised to consult one of the standard anatomy and physiology texts (e.g. Seeley et al., 1995) for a good overview of the subject.

The physiology and radiographic appearance of normal adult bone

An adult long bone, e.g. the humerus, a metacarpal or a phalanx, comprises a shaft that widens out at either end to form articular surfaces that join to other bones. A bony structure comprises cortical (also called compact bone), which forms the strong outer surface of the bone; within the cortex there is cancellous (also known as trabecular) bone, and a central medullary cavity. Cancellous bone is lighter and much less dense than cortical bone, but still contributes to the overall strength of the structure. The spaces within the cancellous bone and the medullary cavity are filled with bone marrow that produces blood cells. Bone tissue itself comprises about one-third organic collagen matrix and two-thirds inorganic mineral salts, calcium and phosphorus.

The outer surface of the cortex of the bone is covered with the *periosteum*. This is tough and fibrous on the outside and continuous with attached tendons and ligaments, but on the inside it is well supplied with blood vessels to provide nutrition, growth and repair. The periosteum covers the entire surface of the bone except at the ends that form part of a joint. In the joint the surface of the bone is covered with hyaline articular cartilage which gives a nearly friction-free surface to allow easy movement of the joint. Neither the periosteum nor hyaline articular cartilage are visible on radiographs, although under certain conditions of disease (e.g. infection) the periosteum does become visible; this is discussed later in this chapter. Throughout the bone matrix there are bone cells, which enable the bone to grow, repair and reshape by laying down new bone and removing unwanted bone during initial skeletal development and following injury.

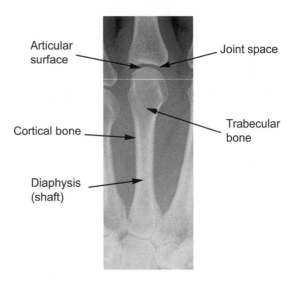

Figure 3.1 The radiographic appearance of an adult metacarpal.

The appearances of the various components of a normal adult bone are shown in a radiograph in Figure 3.1. The shaft of a long bone is known as the *diaphysis* and on the radiograph is seen with a dense (i.e. whiter) rim, which is the outer cortical bone, and a greyer honeycomb-patterned centre representing the trabecular bone. The periosteum is closely applied to the outer surface of the cortical bone and not normally visible on the film. Likewise, the hyaline cartilage which covers the articular ends of the bone is not calcified and therefore is invisible on the radiograph. The joint between two bones is seen as a gap, known as the 'joint space', although in reality this is not a space but two layers of cartilage between which there is a thin film of synovial fluid.

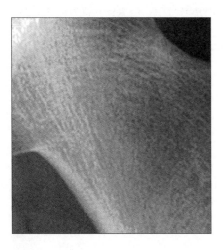

Figure 3.2 This close-up image of a radiograph of the neck of a femur demonstrates the trabecular bone very well. The trabecular patterns align with the weight-bearing stresses that act on the bone, and they give it maximum strength to resist bending and fracture.

Appearance of normal juvenile bone

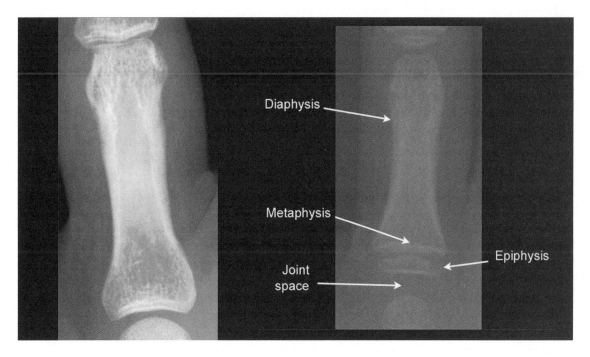

Figure 3.3 Normal adult phalanx (left) and normal immature juvenile phalanx (right).

Most of the long bones develop from a rod of cartilage by a process of *ossification* whereby mineral salts (calcium and phosphorous) are laid down in the cartilaginous matrix (the clavicle is one exception; it ossifies from within a membrane). Cartilage is not visible on the radiograph, so images of the bones of young children will only show the parts of each bone that have ossified. In order for the long bones to grow normally and lengthen in proportion to the overall structure, there is a 'growth plate' at one end of the bone, which is a band or plate of cartilage separating the bone shaft from the *epiphysis* (the term given to the extremities or ends of the bone). With reference to Figure 3.2 (right), the growth plate is seen as a gap close to the end of the long bone. The *metaphysis* is the term given to the growing end of the long bone at the end of the diaphysis, and the bone lengthens from this surface. As the child grows older and the skeleton matures, this gap will close and the epiphysis will fuse with the rest of the shaft. When this fusion is complete, the bone will no longer grow. The appearances of the open epiphyseal plate and the process of fusion can give rise to appearances that mimic a fracture, which must be borne in mind when looking at X-ray films of the immature skeleton. To aid this, it is well worth learning the position and the radiographic appearance of the sites of epiphyses.

Compare the mature and immature phalanges in Figure 3.3. Apart from the separate epiphysis, the joint space itself is more than twice as wide in the immature bone. The cartilage layer is thicker in the juvenile bone, and this has the effect of forming a protective layer around the bone which renders it a little less susceptible to fracture. Thus, an injury which would result in a fracture in an adult may not necessarily do so in a child, and the range of fractures in the skeleton are dependent on age as well as mechanism and force of injury.

Classification of bones and joints

In the appendicular skeleton, the bones encountered are either long bones, short bones or sesamoid bones. Long bones are by far the most numerous, and include the humerus, radius, phalanges, fibula, metatarsals and so on, and range in size from a few millimetres, as in the phalanges of the small toes, to the largest bone in the body: the femur.

The short bones consist of the eight named carpal bones and seven named tarsal bones and are small and irregular in shape. They do not contain bone marrow. Sesamoid bones are normally small rounded bones that form within a tendon in order to resist wear from other neighbouring bone structures. The patella is the largest sesamoid bone, although about 5% of the population have a second smaller sesamoid posteriorly in the knee joint known as the fabella.

The bones, because of their particular function and location and the various tendons and ligaments that attach to them, have a great variety of features such as elevations, holes, projections and so on. Those that are pertinent to the appendicular skeleton are tabulated in Table 3.1.

Table 3.1 Definitions of common bone features (after Gunn, 2002)

Bone feature	Definition	Bone feature	Definition
canal	a bony tunnel	fossa	a wide depression
condyle	a smooth rounded elevation covered in hyaline cartilage at the articulating ends of a long bone	meatus	a narrow passage
		notch	a large groove
		process	a localized projection
crest	a sharp ridge	spine	an elongated process
epicondyle	an elevation above a condyle	sulcus	a groove or furrow
facet	a smooth area covered in hyaline cartilage	trochanter	a large rounded elevation
		trochlea	a pulley-shaped surface
fissure	a narrow slit	tubercle	a small rounded elevation
foramen	a hole	tuberosity	a large rounded elevation

Almost all the joints that are encountered in the appendicular skeleton are *synovial* joints. These are joints between bones where the articulating surfaces are covered by *hyaline cartilage*, which is a smooth substance that reduces friction very efficiently. The joint is encapsulated with a fibrous layer that attaches to the bone surfaces and is lined with a synovial membrane. This membrane secretes synovial fluid that further reduces friction by lubricating the articulating surfaces. The joint is strengthened by tough ligaments that hold the bones in their correct relationship with each other but allow movement of the joint. The degree of free movement depends on the function of the joint, e.g. the shoulder joint can move in almost any direction, whereas the joints between the phalanges of the fingers only allow flexion and extension. In addition to the synovial joints there are some fibrous joints; in particular, there are a few *syndesmoses* where a band or membranous strip of ligaments bind two bones together but still allow a degree of movement. In the appendicular skeleton, the principle syndesmoses are the distal and middle tibio-fibular joints and the radio-ulnar joints. For further information on the classification of bones and joints see Gunn (2002).

Types of fractures and dislocations

There are different ways of classifying a fracture in order to describe the mechanism of injury, the site of fracture and the type and alignment of the fracture. Having a good working knowledge of fracture classification is very useful to those whose role includes diagnosing from radiographs. This enables the concise and accurate description of an injury either in patients' notes or when describing an injury for referral. Table 3.2 lists the important methods used.

Table 3.2 Definitions of fracture types

Feature	Radiographic appearance
Complete	fracture line extends across the bone from one cortex to the other separating the bone into two complete and separate fragments
Greenstick	seen in children, only one cortex is fractured, e.g. distal radial shaft fracture
Torus	again seen in children, with a buckling of the cortex but no break seen
Comminuted	a fracture where there is more than one fracture line that results in at least one separate fragment
Depressed	a portion of bone, normally a joint surface, is forced below the level of the surrounding bone, e.g. depressed tibial plateau fracture
Avulsion	a sudden muscle contraction leading to a piece of bone being pulled off – this is commonly seen in finger injuries and base of fifth metatarsal fracture

Table 3.2 Definitions of fracture types (continued)

Feature	Radiographic appearance
Stress	fractures occurring as a result of repetitive injuries rather than a single event – a cortical break is not always seen but there is a greying of the cortex due to callus formation
Compression/crush	often seen in calcaneal fractures and toes, where the weight of impact crushes the bone
Insufficiency fracture	bone is weakened due to loss of density, typically from osteoporosis – normal activities can cause stress-type fractures, which are seen as locally increased density due to callus formation
Pathological	weaknesses in diseased bone (e.g. cancer) lead to fracture following no or little trauma (e.g. simply turning over in bed)
Compound	there is an open wound that communicates with the fracture site rendering it vulnerable to infection
Dislocation	there is a complete disruption of a joint with no contact between the articular surfaces of the component bones
Subluxation	there is a partial but not complete contact of the articular surfaces of a joint

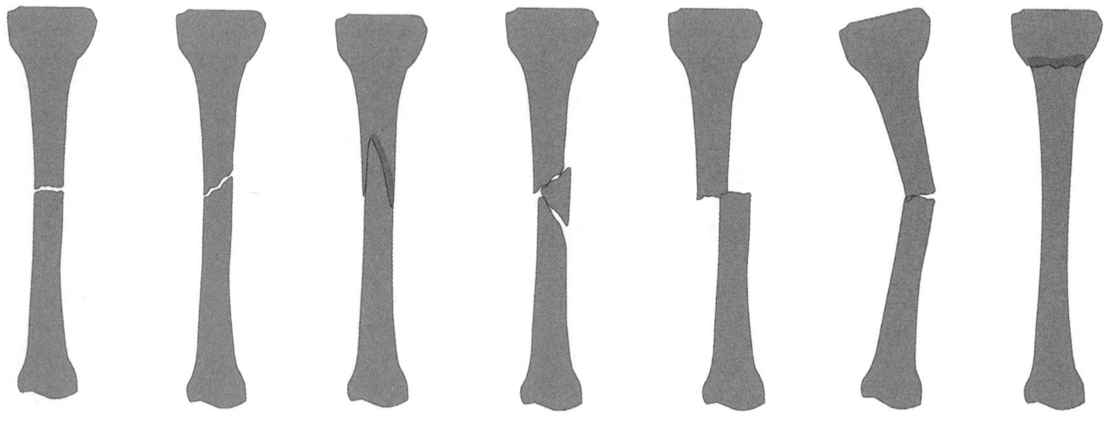

Figure 3.4 Direction and alignment of fractures from left to right: transverse, oblique, spiral, comminuted, displaced angulated and impacted. These seven descriptions, combined appropriately, are sufficient to describe most fractures accurately and relate the seriousness of the injury to a third party.

Juvenile fractures

Fractures of the growing end of a juvenile long bone that involve the growth plate are conventionally described according to the Salter and Harris (1960) classification. Damage to the growth plate and its vulnerable blood supply can affect the subsequent development of the bone, and it is important to describe correctly the injury in question. Figure 3.5 (top left) shows the normal relationship of the epiphysis to the metaphysis. Figure 3.5 (top centre) demonstrates a fracture through the growth plate; no fracture of bone is seen but the epiphysis is shifted from its normal alignment with the shaft (type I). This fracture can be very subtle. Figure 3.5 (top right) is a fracture through the growth plate and through the metaphysis (type II); this is the most common. Figure 3.5 (bottom left) shows a fracture of the growth plate and the epiphysis (type III). Figure 3.5 (bottom centre) shows a fracture of both metaphysis and epiphysis (type IV) and Figure 3.5 (bottom right) demonstrates a compression fracture that closes the growth plate gap by crushing the cartilage (type V). Types I and V, in particular, can be hard to spot. If in doubt, follow-up views can be useful as callus formation is often evident after a delay if a fracture is present. As these fractures heal, there is a risk of bone bridging across the growth plate before the normal age of fusion, and this potentially causes abnormal bone shape and reduction in function.

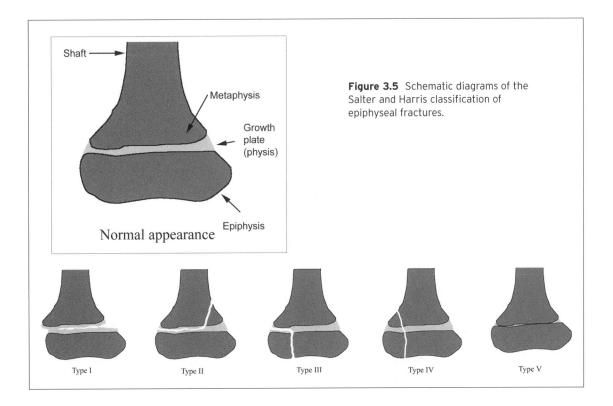

Figure 3.5 Schematic diagrams of the Salter and Harris classification of epiphyseal fractures.

It is rare to see fractures in very young (pre-walking) babies and, if seen, these may be indicative of non-accidental injury (NAI). This is a serious and difficult subject as failure to detect NAI is potentially devastating for that child; however, it is realistically beyond the scope of this book to discuss this issue in any depth; nevertheless the following points may be helpful.

If multiple fractures are seen, particularly at different stages of healing, this would be highly indicative of NAI; however, be aware also that in children aged 2 and above most NAI injuries present only as a single fracture of a long bone. The crucial point is that the presenting injury should fit reasonably with the account from the accompanying adult as to the mechanism of injury and a very careful history should be taken. If there is a suspicion that these are NAIs, a skeletal survey should be done to look for further injuries. However, a skeletal survey for NAI is *never* done as an A&E request; it is done in normal working hours after consultation between the paediatrician, the supervising radiologist and the examining radiographers. Other agencies outside of the hospital environment such as the police and social services may be closely involved in the case. The reader is strongly advised to become familiar with the NAI guidelines in their department, recommended reading includes the section on NAI in Thornton and Gyll (1999), and Hoskote et al. (2003) and Meadow (1997).

The process of fracture healing

Bone is a tissue that is constantly metabolically active, i.e. bone is laid down by bone-producing cells (*osteoblasts*) and is removed by bone-absorbing (*osteoclasts*) cells. These processes are under hormonal control, and in this way the bone is able to respond to physical demands such as weight-bearing or increased activity; it is also able to repair following injury. When a bone fractures, a healing process commences almost immediately that will attempt to repair the damage and restore its mechanical strength and function. Initially, there will be

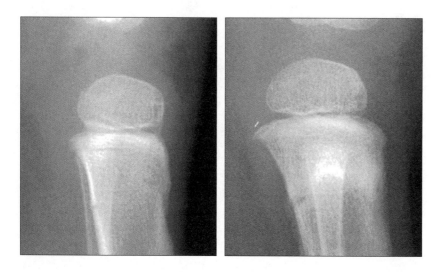

Figure 3.6 Fracture healing. The image on the left was taken on the day of injury and a break in the cortex is just visible at the posterior aspect of the tibia. After eighteen days, the image on the right shows that the cortical break is much less distinct; in addition, there is a denser band of bone across the depth of the tibia indicating increased mineralization as the bone repairs and callus forms.

bleeding at the fracture site from ruptured blood vessels in the bone and a *haematoma* forms. Over the first 24 hours, the haematoma granulates and is invaded by bone-producing cells that generate new bone at the fracture site. This somewhat disorganized local area of new bone is known as a *callus* and at this stage, which is about 7 days post-injury; the evidence of healing will be visible on the radiograph. From this point on, a process of remodelling takes place with a moulding of the new bone by osteoblasts and osteoclasts to restore the original form.

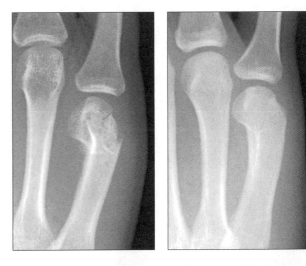

Figure 3.7 The image on the left shows a fractured neck of the fifth metacarpal on the day of injury, while that on the right is over one year post-injury. The angulation of the fracture has not improved but the bone has healed in this position and formed a new cortex. Remodelling and repair has occurred that has replaced the fragmented appearance of the acute injury with a smooth, continuous bone texture.

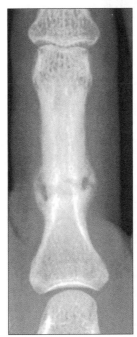
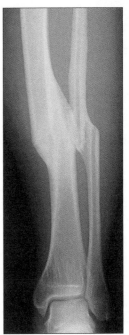

Figure 3.8 The image on the left is a proximal phalanx of the ring finger approximately six weeks post-injury. There is some evidence of the original fracture line; however, there is obvious new bone bridging across the fracture site. A small amount of movement tends to promote callus formation, and it is probable that the finger was not kept completely immobilized during the healing process. The tibia and fibular shaft fractures (right) have healed despite the degree of displacement of the original injury; note the bridging of the fractures with new bone, but the original bone cortex is still clearly visible.

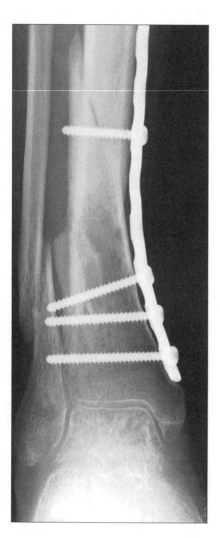

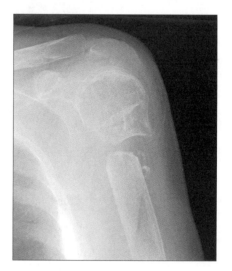

Figure 3.9 Two examples of complications of fracture healing. On the left there has been a surgical fixation of a comminuted fracture of the distal tibia and fibula. The bone texture proximal to the fracture is normal with a reasonable thickness of cortex apparent, whereas the bone distal to the fracture has become demineralized resulting in a thinned cortex and much less dense bone. In addition, there is no evidence of callus formation around the fracture, indicating non-union. In fact, although surgical intervention will immobilize and stabilize an unstable fracture, callus formation is promoted by a degree of movement at the fracture site. Fractures immobilized surgically may show very little evidence of callus formation because there is no movement owing to the rigidity of the repair. The image on the right demonstrates a long-term failure of a fracture to unite. This fracture of the proximal humerus has never united and resulted in the well-rounded and smooth appearance of the fracture ends. In fact, this appearance is known as a *pseudoarthrosis* as there may well be movement at the site which mimics that of a joint.

Appearance of abnormal or diseased bone

It is important in the A&E/MIU environment to expect the unexpected. Although most referrals for X-ray will be for an acute injury, occasionally non-traumatic disease and lesions that are not due to injury but to another, possibly sinister, cause will be seen on the resulting films. However, there are many conditions that may appear on the radiograph as unusual or mimicking disease but which are simply variations in normal bone. It is vital that anyone using radiographs as a diagnostic tool has the skill to detect not only the acute injury for which the X-ray would have been requested but also to recognize a change from the normal bone appearance, which may be due to a pathological process such as arthritis, infection or cancerous tumour. The purpose of this section is to introduce the reader to some of the radiographic appearances that are due to such diseases in order that the abnormality might be referred and followed up appropriately. It is not intended, by any means, to be a comprehensive account of all pathological disease processes affecting bone, but to give an insight into some of the more common appearances likely to be encountered. Further reading on the subject is advised and by Clyde Helms (1994) is a very accessible and concise introduction and definitely worth investing in.

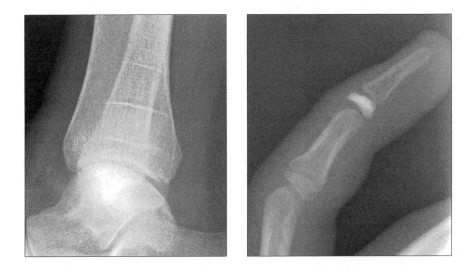

Figure 3.10 The left-hand image is of 'Harris' lines in the distal tibia caused by an interruption to normal growth of the bone in childhood, normally due to illness. The bone stops lengthening but dense mineral salts continue to be laid down thus increasing the density of the bone at this point and giving the horizontal thin white bands seen. The right-hand image shows a 'bright' epiphysis in the distal phalanx of a little finger. This appearance is unusual but is not pathological, as it is caused by a profusion of dense cortical bone in the epiphysis, although the appearance of the epiphysis of the middle phalanx is more usual. Neither of these conditions would be considered abnormal or pathological, but, if you are ever unsure of an appearance on a film, get an expert radiological opinion.

Features of abnormal bone

Table 3.3, overleaf, lists the common features of bone diseases that you should look out for when interpreting a radiograph. These should be incorporated in the scan of every radiograph in order to detect non-fracture-type lesions and diseases. This is a very simplified list, and large books have been written that concentrate on diagnosis of tumours and other diseases on radiographs. It is a specialized and expert field that cannot be learnt quickly. Examples of these are seen throughout the rest of this chapter.

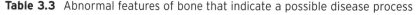

Table 3.3 Abnormal features of bone that indicate a possible disease process

Feature	Radiographic appearance
periosteal reaction	the bone cortex may be thickened or with a double line appearance – this may be solid or wispy and interrupted
bone shape	lesions may be expansile causing the bone to bulge – bone may be deformed in shape
bone cortex	can be thinned or destroyed
trabecular bone pattern	bone texture may be destroyed with a moth-eaten or permeative appearance, or there may be increased bone density
lesion boundary	'zone of transition' may be sharp and narrow or ill-defined and broad – there may be a sclerotic, dense border or no defined border
adjacent tissues	extension into adjacent tissues or soft-tissue mass seen
site of lesion	centre or edge of bone, abutting a joint or epiphysis, solitary or multiple lesions

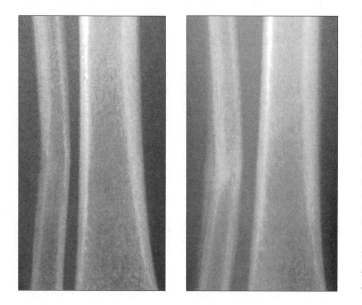

Figure 3.11 Periosteal reaction in the fibular shaft. Periosteal reaction is an important feature of many bone diseases and conditions, and in some cases the earliest radiographic indication of an abnormality. The image on the left shows the fibular shaft of a 2-year-old boy who refused to walk. The bone appears to be bent slightly towards the tibia. The image on the right is of the same region of bone fourteen days later. The angulation is similar but the outer cortex is now thickened when compared with the original image. In fact, there is a slight lifting of the periosteum seen on the original image, which appears as a subtle double line of cortex. This is one example of periosteal reaction. The abnormality in this case is a *plastic bowing fracture* where no fracture line or cortical break is seen but the shape of the bone is abnormal and the fracture is confirmed by the periosteal reaction.

Degenerative joint disease

The joints between the bones that allow movement are susceptible to a range of diseases, the most common of which is osteoarthritis; this may be primary – the degenerative ageing process of joints – or secondary as a result of previous injury or other disease condition of the affected joint. *Arthritis* is a term that also includes other inflammatory or infectious joint diseases such as rheumatoid arthritis, gout or septic arthritis. Diagnosis of these conditions is not normally reached simply from plain X-rays but from further diagnostic tests; however, images of osteoarthritis are included as this is seen in many patients who have X-rays and the features on the images can be very marked.

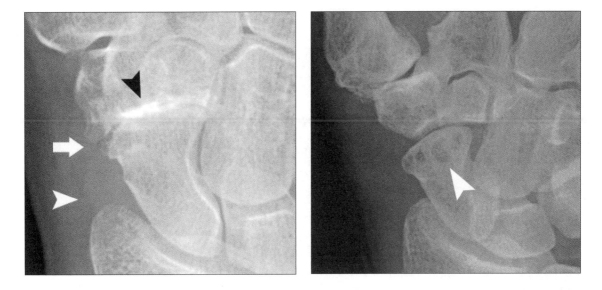

Figure 3.12 These two detailed radiographs of the scaphoid and associated joints of two elderly patients show some typical changes seen due to degenerative joint disease – osteoarthritis – including loss of joint space and sclerosis of the bone adjacent to the eroded joint (black arrowhead, left). There is an overgrowth of the margins of the bone (white arrow, left) known as osteophytosis. There is also a bulge in the soft tissues seen (white arrowhead, left), which is indicative of a joint effusion. Occasionally, subchondral cysts are seen; this occurs when synovial fluid from the joint penetrates the cortex and forms a cyst just adjacent to the joint margin (white arrowhead, right).

In addition, there is a loss of bone density with thinning of the cortex and one or two small lucent regions seen in the distal radial shaft indicating a loss of bone density, or osteoporosis. Osteoporosis is most often seen in post-menopausal women and renders the bone brittle and susceptible to fracture. Strictly speaking, however, the term *osteoporosis* is not used when describing a loss of bone density seen on a radiograph as it is impossible to distinguish between that and osteomalacia (*osteomalacia* is a disease of abnormal bone matrix rather than simply a loss of mineral bone content). Instead, the term *osteopoenia* is used, and this will often be encountered in radiological reports that describe a reduction in bone density.

Infection

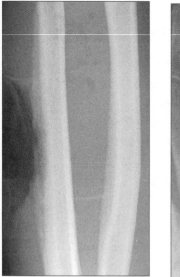 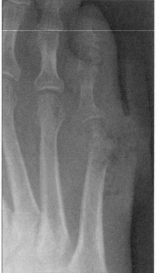

Figure 3.13 Bone infection. The image on the left is of a young intravenous drug abuser with a large soft-tissue abscess in the forearm. The infection has tracked to the bone causing chronic periostitis with the thickened cortical appearance. The image on the right is of a middle-aged diabetic man with chronic foot ulcers. No periostitis is seen but there is a loss of the normal bone cortex of the fifth metacarpal head. Infection does not usually show on plain X-ray films for at least fourteen days; so a normal appearance does not mean that there is no bone involvement. Bear in mind also that the appearance of bone infection is very variable. These are just two examples, but there are many others, and infection can mimic other bone abnormalities. Always get an expert opinion.

Osteochondritis

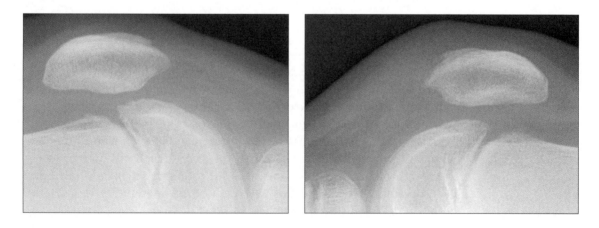

Figure 3.14 Osteochondritis of the lower pole of the patella. This is known as Sindig-Larsen-Johanssen disease and is one of a range of named examples of osteochondritis. The patella shown on the left is normal but that on the right of the same 9-year-old boy is fragmented at its distal pole, and there is considerable soft-tissue swelling overlying this region. Osteochondritis is characterized by pain and swelling without necessarily any single traumatic origin. It is more common in boys and may be due to excessive demands on still-immature bone structures. Other sites include the tibial tuberosity, femoral head, capitellum (capitulum in some textbooks) of the elbow, lunate, navicular and the second metatarsal head. If seen, get an expert opinion in order to exclude other causes such as infection and for any necessary treatment. There are also normal variants that can mimic the appearance of osteochondritis. Reference to Keats's *Atlas of Normal Röntgen Variants* is also useful as well as correlation with the clinical signs.

Benign cystic lesions

Figure 3.15 This is a fibrous cortical defect (left and detail right) – also called a non-ossifying fibroma – which is a region of abnormally developed bone. They are seen commonly in the distal tibia in young people and normally heal by the mid-twenties. Note that it comprises a less dense region of bone which expands slightly beyond the normal boundary. There is a slightly dense (sclerotic) border separating the lesion from the normal trabecular pattern. A residual, slightly denser, region of bone is often seen following healing.

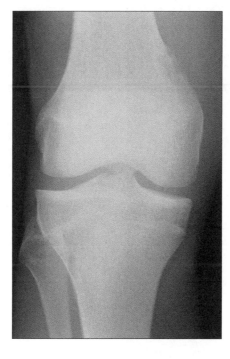
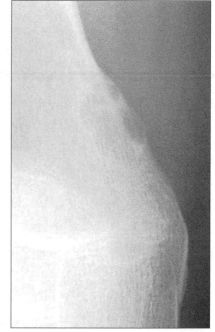

Figure 3.16 This is a simple bone cyst in a 9-year-old boy (left) and when 11 years old (right). Note the bubbly appearance with a dense sclerotic boundary and minimal expansion of the bone. It does not cross the epiphyseal plate. In the later film, there is more normal bone between the cystic lesion and the proximal end of the tibia. This is because the bone has lengthened over the intervening two years with the effect that the cyst appears to have moved down the bone whereas in actual fact the bone has grown above it.

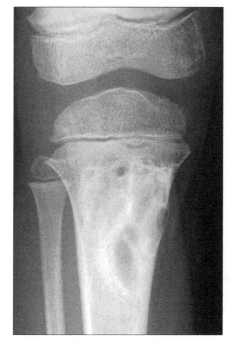
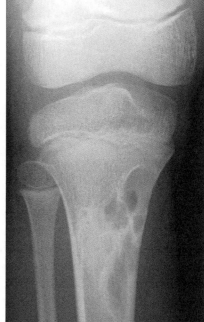

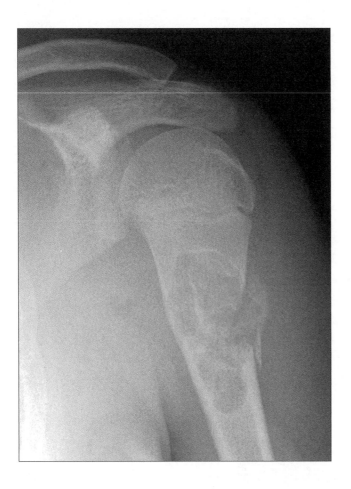

Figure 3.17 Another simple bone cyst. However, this time it has severely weakened the humerus, resulting in a pathological fracture. There is a risk of repeated fracture with this size of bone cyst, and surgical intervention may be undertaken under certain circumstances to encourage a more rapid healing.

Cancerous bone tumours

Bone, as in any other living tissue, is susceptible to invasion by tumour. This may be a primary bone tumour, secondary spread from adjacent soft tissues or metastatic spread from a tumour distant to the site of appearance. There are signs on plain X-rays as to the type of tumour that might be present; however, it is well beyond the scope of this book to go into any great detail. Suffice it to say that any bone lesions noted on a radiograph as an incidental finding should always be followed up by an expert opinion, referral and further diagnostic tests as necessary. Never assume that an appearance is benign or insignificant; there are many examples of non-threatening lesions that can have almost exactly the same appearance as a malignant process, and the differentiation of these should be left to others. As a guide, the most common primary tumours that lead to bone metastases are lung, breast and prostate.

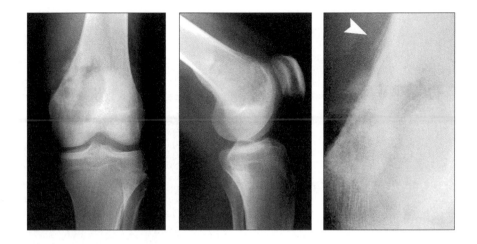

Figure 3.18 Osteosarcoma. This is an aggressive, malignant tumour of the lower femur in a 17-year-old boy who had unexplained pain in the knee. The main radiographic features that should immediately raise concern are the wispy new bone formation seen extending into the soft tissues, a triangle of raised periosteum separating normal bone cortex from destroyed cortex – known as 'Codman's triangle', see arrowhead on detail view below – and an infiltrative moth-eaten appearance in the main bone without a dense border indicating rapid advance of abnormal bone.

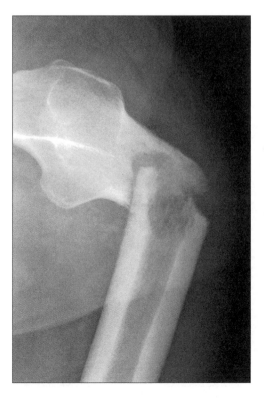

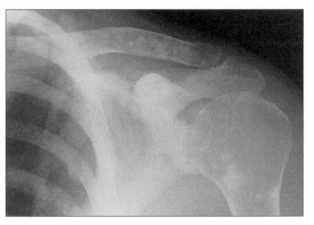

Figure 3.19 Bone metastasis. The image on the left is of a pathological fracture through a metastatic deposit in the proximal femur. Tumour has destroyed the bone tissue leaving it considerably weaker – a stress such as an awkward stumble, which would normally be resisted by healthy bone, has led to a complete fracture through the femoral shaft. The image on the right is of advanced bone metastasis from a primary prostate tumour. In contrast to the lytic (i.e. bone-removing) tumour in the previous example, the appearances are of multiple dense lesions. Note that there are deposits throughout all the bones demonstrated, including the ribs.

Figure 3.20 This extraordinary appearance in the tibia of a 76-year-old man is due to Paget's disease. This is occasionally seen: look out for a very coarsened trabecular appearance with expansion of the bone. The fibula is unaffected but has a tethering effect at either end of the tibia preventing it lengthening; this has resulted in the bowing appearance seen.

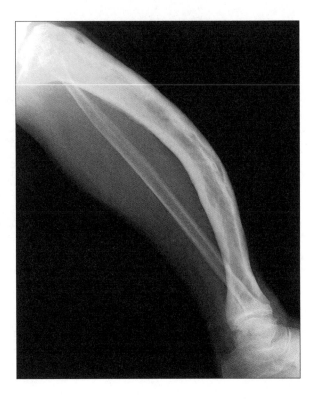

Developmental abnormalities

In summary, it is important to examine the X-ray films you request carefully not only for the mechanical fractures that you might be expecting but also for abnormalities in bone texture that might indicate a pathological disease process. Always get bone lesions checked and don't jump to conclusions regarding the origin. Remember, an experienced radiologist will always give a list of possible diagnoses from the most common and likely to the rarer, but still possible, cause that must be investigated and excluded by further imaging or other diagnostic test. After you have browsed through the following anatomical chapters, it will be worth rereading this chapter to compare the mechanical fracture-type abnormalities seen with the disease processes presented here.

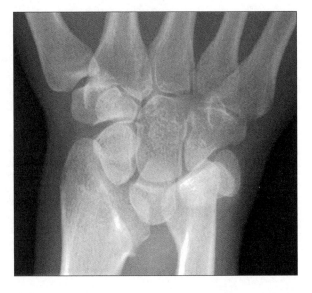

Figure 3.21 This peculiar-looking appearance of the wrist is due to Madelung's deformity. The medial aspect of the radial epiphyses has fused prematurely. This has stopped the bone lengthening at this point, whereas the unaffected part of the bone has kept growing. When the entire epiphysis finally fused, the radial articular surface has this characteristic acute angulation, which has allowed the carpal bones to wedge into the triangular space that has resulted. This is one example of a developmental abnormality that just occasionally appears on a radiograph, and there are countless others.

Part II

The Radiology of the
Anatomical Regions

Introduction to the anatomical chapters

The aim of this section is to cover some general aspects and principles of radiographic interpretation that are applicable to all plain film examinations – specific points for regional injuries are dealt with under each anatomical chapter.

Recognition of abnormalities comes with repeat exposure, but utilizing a systematic approach will guide you while you build up your experience and help identify more-subtle findings. However, a good knowledge of the normal anatomy is a pre-requisite; no system can replace this. A useful and commonly used system is the AABCS (Touquet et al., 1995):

Assessment of film
Alignment
Bones
Cartilage
Soft tissues

Assessment of film

Before commencing interpretation, it is important to make sure that the viewing conditions are optimal. Radiographs are best viewed in subdued lightning on a light box that has a bright light (or use a lamp) for viewing soft tissues. Assessing a radiograph by holding it up to the ceiling light is inexcusably poor practice and will result in not identifying some abnormalities, especially subtle ones. A magnifying glass is useful when conventional film is used. If you are using digital X-ray technology, ensure that you are able to use the features of the viewing software such as magnification and brightness and contrast adjustment. However, avoid over-magnifying; this tends to create apparent fractures out of the most insignificant ripple in the bone pattern.

Next, look at the quality of the film: is it under- or over-exposed? A good exposure should demonstrate the bony trabeculae as well as the soft tissues. Under-exposure will produce insufficient bone detail, while over-exposure will obliterate the soft tissues. Sometimes, it is useful to stand back a bit to view the radiograph as a whole, rather than focusing immediately on the suspected abnormality. Subtleties are often spotted this way. If you see an obvious abnormality, your suspicion for a second abnormality should be raised, especially if the clinical examination revealed a second query. Reassess the radiograph systematically covering all areas, and positively rule out other abnormalities.

A very important early step in the assessment of a radiograph is to ensure that all the details of the examination are correct. The examining radiographer should have ensured that all the patient demographic details (name, gender, date of birth etc.) are accurate, but whoever is interpreting the radiograph must do the same. Particularly in film-based departments it is frighteningly easy for a radiograph to be slipped into the incorrect packet – but digital images can contain incorrect information as well. Check *every* film for correct patient identification.

Check that the left or right markers are on the radiograph and are correct and that you understand the orientation of the projections that were done. If the marker is not what you expect, is it because the wrong side was examined or because the wrong marker was applied to the film? The radiographer should check with the patient which is the affected side, but mistakes can still happen, and patients do not always speak up when a mistake is being made.

The 'rule of two' is applicable to most examinations: two views and two joints. Some abnormalities are only visible in one view, therefore a second view at 90° to the first is taken. Examples of such injuries are included in the subsequent chapters. Likewise, certain bones (e.g. radius and ulna) are held together with strong ligaments – an angulated fracture to one of these bones results in a relative shortening, and consequent dislocation, of the other. The clinical examination of any bones must include 'joint above

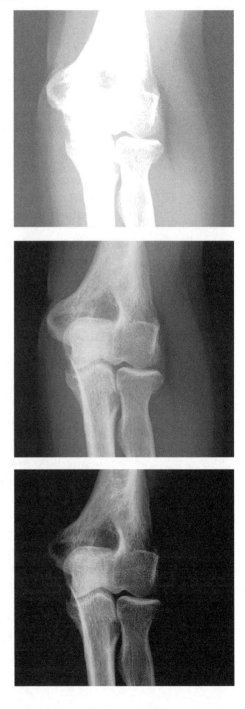

Figure II Three exposures of the same image. These images have been altered to give an idea of over- and under-exposure. The top image is underexposed The soft-tissue planes are seen well but there is no bone detail as insufficient penetration of the bone has occurred. The centre image is a good exposure: the soft tissues are visible and the bone detail such as the cortex and trabecular pattern are well differentiated. The bottom image is over-exposed. All of the soft tissues and some of the thinner bone regions have been obliterated. The fracture of the radial head is best seen on the central image.

and below' to prevent missing these injuries, and these must be X-rayed if clinically indicated.

Alignment

An X-ray examination can be looked at as a collection of individual bones, and scrutinized as such, whereas in reality a joint should be viewed as a single entity made up of several components. The relationship between the individual bones in a joint must be assessed in order to detect dislocations, subluxations and joint instability due to ligamentous disruption. Look at each bone individually, and then look at the whole structure. Where appropriate, we have included useful alignment lines and signs for each anatomical region in order to help detect subtle dislocations and fractures.

Bones

Each bone should be traced and examined for a break in the cortex and for evidence of unusual angulation that might indicate a greenstick or plastic bowing fracture. Examine the trabecular pattern very carefully. As discussed in Chapter 3, the trabeculae are the thin plates of bone that make up the cancellous bone matrix which is within the outer shell of cortical bone. The trabeculae are arranged in a pattern that aligns with the mechanical stress placed on the bone. Disruption to the trabecular pattern can indicate a subtle or impacted fracture or it could indicate a pathological process such as infection or tumour that has invaded the bone – a *lytic* lesion. The bone cortex should also be checked for abnormal thinning or destruction and for periosteal reaction.

Cartilage

Cartilage, ligaments and tendons are not seen on a radiograph unless they have become calcified for some reason. Consequently, we tend to refer to the gaps between the bones on a radiograph as a *joint space*, whereas in reality there is no space: the articular surfaces of the bones are lined with hyaline articular cartilage. Abnormally narrowed joint spaces indicate a disease process, most commonly degenerative disease such as osteoarthritis. Fractures that involve the joint are significant as the function of that joint can be affected, in the short term, if the fracture heals unsatisfactorily and affects the joint movements, and in the long term if arthritic changes secondary to the injury further damage the joint causing pain and loss of function.

Soft tissues

Soft-tissue planes can demonstrate swelling, which is a useful pointer to a possible underlying injury. There are several 'fat pads', most notably the elbow, which if abnormal can be highly suggestive of fracture. A classic soft-tissue sign is a joint effusion where trauma (or possibly infection) causes an abnormal amount of fluid to collect within the joint capsule causing it to bulge, contrasting with the surrounding muscular soft tissues. Fat, fluid or air interfaces appear well on a radiograph and can give clues to otherwise occult (unseen) injuries. Lastly, don't forget to exclude penetrating foreign bodies such as metal or glass, particularly with an open wound.

A note on radiographic 'projections'

There are common terms to describe the angle or direction of the X-ray beam used (the radiographic projection). Ideally, two views at right angles are taken and a term is given to each of the views based on the direction of the X-ray beam in relation to the normal anatomical position. The projections listed below are most often used; however, there are many others (see Glossary).

antero-posterior (AP)	the beam passes from the front to the back of the patient
postero-anterior (PA)	the beam passes from the back to the front of the patient
dorsi-plantar or dorsi-palmer (DP)	similar to the above but refers to the foot and hand, respectively
lateral	a sideways view, although there are several named variations when the projection is not truly at right angles to the midline of the patient
oblique	neither straight on nor sideways, the oblique view is a second view where a lateral does not demonstrate the bony anatomy adequately due to superimposition

Textbooks and other resources

It is exceptionally useful to have to hand certain textbooks to aid your image interpretation. If you ever look in a radiologist's office or reporting room, you will see many different texts and tomes that aid in X-ray diagnosis. For plain film reporting, make sure you have a copy of 'Keats (1996). This is a hugely useful (but expensive) textbook that has thousands of images of normal variants in the skeleton that appear to be fractures. Try and get your department to buy a copy. Secondly, have a good orthopaedic radiology textbook. We like *Orthopaedic Radiology* by Adam Greenspan (2000); there is so much useful information on normal anatomy, fractures and pathological bone diseases. It is a hefty book (with a hefty price) but invaluable. A good orthopaedic management textbook is also useful as you decide how to deal with the various injuries that you encounter. We find MacRae (1999), Dandy and Edwards (2003) and Wardrope and English (1998) particularly helpful.

On the Internet, Amersham Health (http://www.amershamhealth. com/) has a very good online medical encyclopaedia that gives concise information on bone pathologies and includes example radiographs.

Chapter 4

The shoulder and proximal humerus

Review of core anatomy

The shoulder is in practice often seen as one joint (the gleno-humeral joint), but the actual shoulder girdle is made up of four joints, which must all be identified in order to correctly interpret a radiograph:

- gleno-humeral joint
- acromio-clavicular joint
- sterno-clavicular joint
- scapulo-humeral joint

The head of the humerus sits on a thick anatomical neck and has two bony prominences known as the greater and lesser tuberosities (see Figure 4.3), which are the insertion point for several muscles. The humerus then narrows to form the shaft and it is at this point that the surgical neck is identified. The scapula sits on the posterior chest wall and can be described as triangular in shape with a neck, body and spine (see Figure 4.3). Trace very carefully around the entire scapula, including the acromion and the apex of the scapula which may be hard to follow when projected against the lungs and ribs. Most of the scapula is difficult to see on the anterior aspect of a radiograph, as the ribs are superimposed, except the lateral aspect where the glenoid cavity can be identified (see Figure 4.1). The uppermost lateral aspect of the scapula terminates in a bony prominence called the *acromion process*, which connects the anterior and posterior of the shoulder. It articulates with the lateral end of the clavicle (Figure 4.3). Medially to the acromion on the superior border of the scapula is a 'hook/beak' process known as the *coracoid process* (Figure 4.3), which serves as an attachment for several muscles and ligaments.

The clavicle is the bony structure lying subcutaneously on the anterior chest wall. It articulates medially with the sternum and has three main functions (Moore, 1992):

- acts as a brace keeping the upper limb free from the trunk to facilitate maximum freedom
- attachment for muscles
- enables forces to be transmitted from the upper limb to the axial skeleton

The gleno-humeral joint is a 'ball and socket' joint with a large head of humerus and a relatively shallow glenoid fossa (approximately one-third of that of the humerus) which is deepened by a cartilaginous ring known as the *glenoid labrum* (see Figure 4.1). The overall effect is a highly mobile joint in which stability is compromised. It is more or less entirely dependent on the surrounding muscles (in particular the rotator cuff), ligaments and capsular tissues for stability. The gleno-humeral joint obtains some support from the gleno-humeral ligaments, although the main stabilizers are the four rotator cuff muscles that all arise in the scapula region with tendon termination in the proximal humerus:

- supraspinatus: shoulder abduction
- infraspinatus and teres minor: lateral rotation of the shoulder
- subcularis: medial rotation

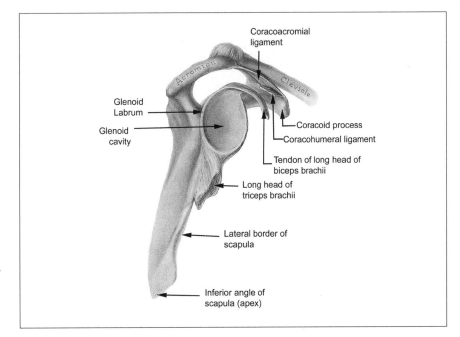

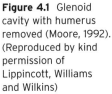

Figure 4.1 Glenoid cavity with humerus removed (Moore, 1992). (Reproduced by kind permission of Lippincott, Williams and Wilkins)

Standard projections

AP and either axial or lateral scapula

Additional projections

angled-up clavicle
acromio-clavicular joints

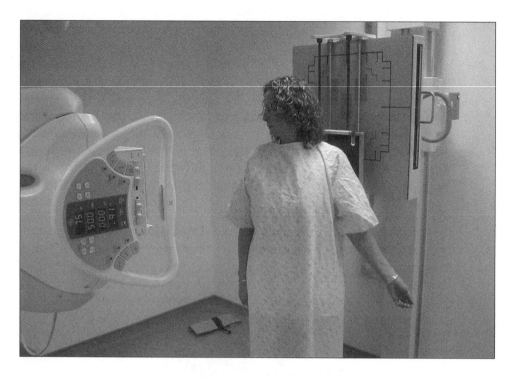

Figure 4.2 For this projection, the patient stands or sits with the cassette supported behind the shoulder and the arm held with the palm facing forward. If the shoulder only is being examined, about one-third to one-half of the humeral shaft is included. If the whole of the humerus is of interest, the entire shaft is included with the elbow joint.

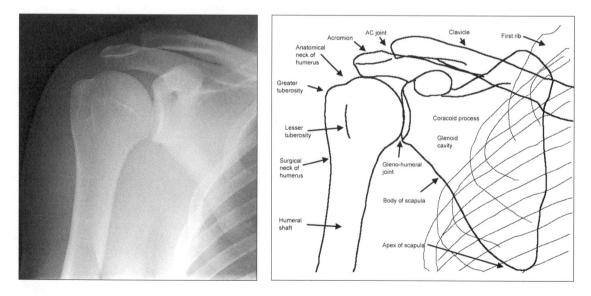

Figure 4.3 The AP shoulder radiograph (left) and outline diagram with anatomical annotation (right).

Trace the borders of all the bones, with reference to Figure 4.3, and check that the greater tuberosity is intact as these can be very subtle fractures. Trace very carefully around the entire scapula, including the spine leading to the acromion and the apex, which may be hard to follow when projected against the lungs and ribs. Follow the clavicle along its entire length and check that the lower outer border aligns with the lower border of the acromion – the acromio-clavicular joint. When you are satisfied that there are no fractures or dislocations in the shoulder itself, look at the rest of the anatomy on the film – is there a rib fracture and can you see lung markings extending to the chest margin?

The humeral head should appear asymmetrical with the greater tuberosity seen in profile. If the humeral head appears symmetrical (often called a 'light bulb' appearance), do not immediately assume that there is a joint abnormality. Check that the view was not taken with the arm internally rotated – often because the joint was examined with the arm still in the sling – as this will give a similar appearance. The enlocated joint will usually demonstrate an overlap between the humeral head and the glenoid cavity – this is often called the *crescent sign* – see Figure 4.4.

Figure 4.4 Radiograph of the glenoid and humeral head with schematic diagram. The crescent sign (the dark-grey crescent shown in the schematic diagram) is caused by the overlapping articular surfaces of the glenoid and humeral head. This, together with the congruity of the joint lines, shows that the humeral head is located within the glenoid. To be absolutely sure, however, a second view is required.

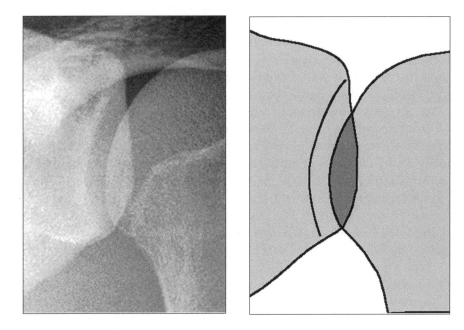

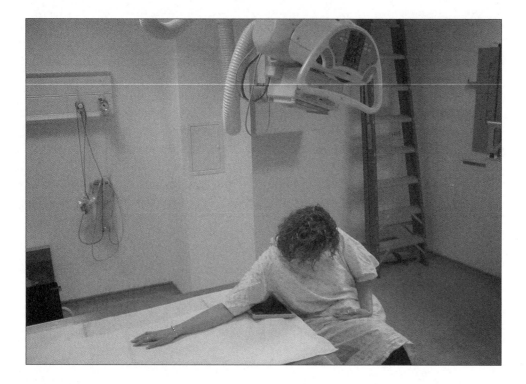

Figure 4.5 Positioning the patient for an axial shoulder view. This position is rarely achievable if the patient has a dislocation or severe fracture.

The axial view (Figure 4.6) is one of the two second views that may be provided, and both seem to cause difficulty in interpretation whereas logically neither should be any more difficult to interpret than the AP view. The key is to orientate yourself with the anatomy by realizing how the projection was obtained. The patient sits sideways at the X-ray table and leans with the affected arm over the table top. The cassette is placed on the table beneath the axilla and the beam is directed from above the patient's shoulder. Note that the coracoid process projects forward; therefore, if you are looking at a right shoulder, physically rotate the film so that the coracoid does project forward and the humeral shaft projects to the right. It will then be much easier to identify the glenoid and confirm that the gleno-humeral joint is located. Usually, however, if there is a humeral fracture or joint dislocation, the patient will be in too much pain to position satisfactorily for this projection and the alternative lateral scapula view will be preferred.

This view also causes difficulties with interpretation; however, familiarity with the anatomy of the projection will clarify the problem. This view is usually taken with the patient standing and facing obliquely towards the X-ray cassette, which is supported in a vertical

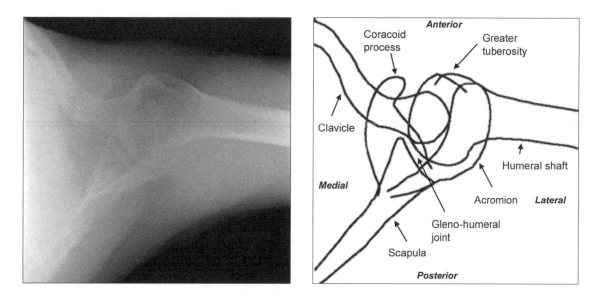

Figure 4.6 The axial view and a schematic outline. The patient sits sideways at the X-ray table and leans over the cassette with the arm extended. In the case of dislocation or humeral fracture, this position is almost impossible to achieve, owing to the patient's discomfort, and an alternative view will normally be done.

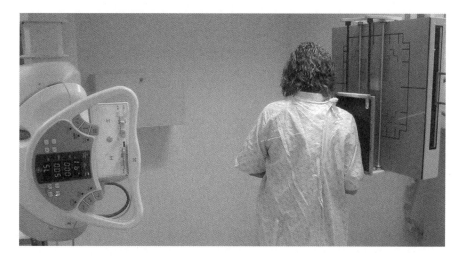

Figure 4.7 Positioning for lateral scapula ('Y' or 'Mercedes') view.

holder. The patient leans towards the cassette so that the humeral head and shaft is in contact with the cassette and the blade of the scapula is perpendicular to it. The X-ray beam is directed at the patient's scapula; the projection is therefore PA. The arm of the affected side can be supported in a sling or by the unaffected hand, i.e. internally rotated. This view demonstrates the blade of the scapula well and is the required second view if a scapular fracture is suspected.

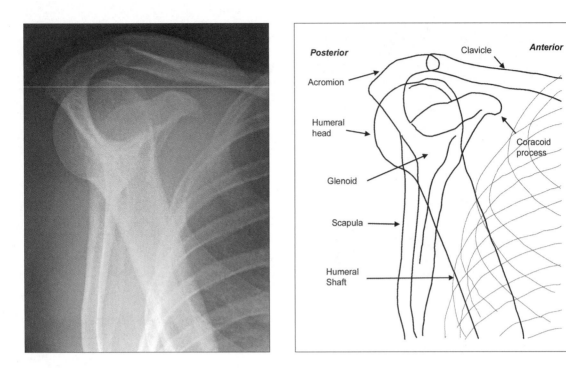

Figure 4.8 Lateral scapula radiograph and a schematic outline. The patient sits or stands obliquely to the X-ray cassette with the affected shoulder touching the cassette.

Again, the coracoid process projects anteriorly and towards the ribs. The glenoid cavity is seen *en face* at the centre of a 'Y' formed by the coracoid and acromion processes with the blade of the scapula forming the shaft of the 'Y'. The humeral head should overlie the glenoid with the humeral shaft projecting downwards and superimposed over the blade of the scapula. The ribs are anterior to the scapula so the direction of a dislocation can be worked out: with the humeral head towards or overlying the ribs, the dislocation is anterior; away from the ribs it has to be posterior.

If the patient is unable to stand, an AP version of this view is possible with the patient sitting on a trolley, but the result is generally less satisfactory due to magnification and distortion. However, it is still useful to confirm or exclude a dislocation. If a humeral shaft fracture is suspected, the PA lateral scapula to include the entire humeral shaft and elbow joint is required.

In high-energy-transfer injuries, such as a fall from a height or RTAs, the cervical spine must be examined and/or immobilized as required. In the absence of a cervical spine injury, check full active neck movements (Wardrope and English, 1998). The elbow must also be routinely examined.

Clinical examination

The shoulder has an extensive supply of nerves arising from the neck into the axilla called the *brachial plexus* formed by branches from C5 to C8 and T1 (Moore, 1992). The branches divide and re-unite in various patterns, but eventually form three main cords (lateral, medial and posterior) in the axilla around the axillary artery. The axillary nerve arises from here and wraps around the back of the humerus. The ulnar, median and radial nerves are all terminal branches of these cords (Moore, 1992; Dean and Pegington, 1996). Any examination of the shoulder must include testing of the axillary nerve, by touching the so-called 'regimental badge' (deltoid insertion). This must be followed by testing of the ulnar, median and radial nerves. Finally, check distal pulses and compare both sides.

Look

Observe the patient from the front, side and back with clothing removed. Compare both sides. How is the posture? Is the patient holding their arm close to the body (adducted) or protecting the arm while walking? Note any area of obvious deformity, swelling, bruising, asymmetry and redness/discoloration. Is the skin intact or can you see bones protruding or lying tight against the skin? How is the patient generally? Distressed with pain? If so, ensure they have adequate analgesia before proceeding.

Feel

First, feel the skin temperature and compare with the other side. Is it cold, hot, clammy? Gently but firmly palpate all anatomical structures to identify the point of maximum tenderness, from the neck, then sterno-clavicular joint throughout clavicle, AC joint, scapula and head of humerus to the elbow. Start your palpation away from the area of injury to gain the patient's trust, moving systematically and purposely towards the site of injury.

Move

Movements should be assessed both actively and passively. However, this may not always be possible in the acutely injured shoulder. As a general rule, the following structures are being assessed during movement:

- active: muscle, bone, joint, tendon
- passive: joints and bones
- resisted: muscle and tendon strength/integrity

There are several specific tests that can be used to identify particular muscles/ligaments injuries, but essentially the shoulder girdle has five main movements:

- flexion (forward): 0°–180°
- extension: 0°–45°
- abduction: 0°-170°
- internal and external rotation: 0°–70°

Most injuries are detectable on the standard AP view; the exceptions are some subtle clavicular fractures, occasionally a posterior gleno-humeral dislocation and some scapular fractures. The principle of two views therefore still applies in order not to miss less obvious abnormalities. The film shown in Figure 4.9 is interesting; no fracture is seen but there is a thin lucent line that is congruent with the articular surfaces of the gleno-humeral joint. This is known as the *gas* or *vacuum sign* as it is caused by a small amount of gas – hence the relative lucency – within the joint and seems to be more common in teenagers. It is a useful sign to look for as it is indicative of two points: first the joint has undergone significant stress or trauma in order for the gas to appear and, secondly, it is not dislocated as the gas lies between the articular surfaces of the joint. The mechanism for the generation of this gas or vacuum is not fully understood; nevertheless, it is a useful sign to watch for on every shoulder radiograph.

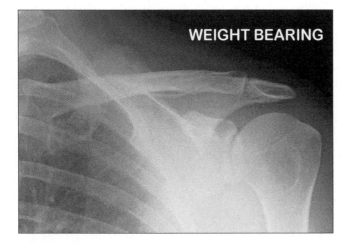

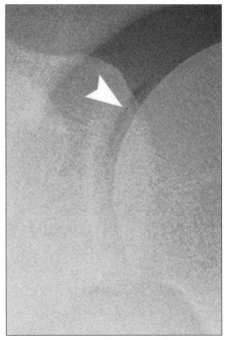

Figure 4.9 Vacuum phenomenon. The thin lucent line seen in the gleno-humeral joint (white arrowhead, detail view) is either a gas, possibly nitrogen, or a vacuum depending on which journal you read. Nevertheless, it is a useful indicator of joint stress and also excludes a dislocation.

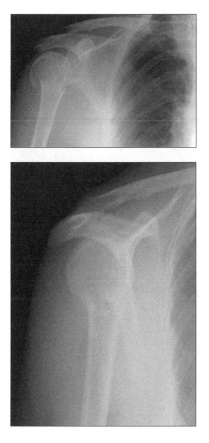

Fractures of the proximal humerus

Commonly seen in the older patient, these fractures are often impacted or comminuted and may be associated with greater tuberosity avulsion fractures, caused by rupture of the supraspinatus tendon. The mechanism of injury is usually through a fall onto the outstretched hand, a fall onto the shoulder or a direct blow. The patient will often support the affected arm by holding it in adduction. Obvious deformities are rare as the humerus is well splinted by numerous muscles, but if present are usually associated with severe displacement/angulation. Swelling may be diffuse, owing to gravity, and bruising extensive (noticeable after a few hours). There is localized tenderness over the proximal end of the humerus. Neurovascular assessment is essential as displaced fractures carry a risk of damage to nerves and blood vessels from sharp bone ends. All movements of the shoulder are grossly restricted due to pain.

Figure 4.10 Surgical neck of humerus fracture (top) and detail view (bottom). Note that the denser, overlapping region of the fracture site indicates a degree of impaction. The lateral scapula does not show a posterior dislocation; the humeral head is seen thrown slightly posterior due to slightly off-lateral positioning.

Figure 4.11 Another example of a surgical neck of humerus fracture after a fall (left) and detail view (right). Note the detached fracture fragment lying inferior to the glenoid and that the humeral head is subluxed inferiorly. Look carefully and you will see a lipohaemarthrosis within the joint capsule (white arrowhead, detail view). This is where fat is floating on blood and creating a fluid/fluid interface seen as a line separating the fat (less dense) from the blood (relatively more dense). This is not often seen in the shoulder, but it is almost always seen in the knee in the presence of a fracture within the joint capsule. This extra fluid within the joint capsule has forced the humeral head inferiorly.

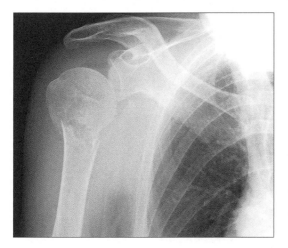

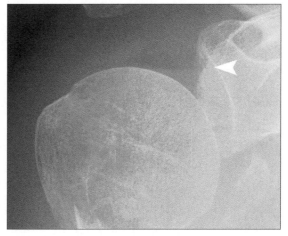

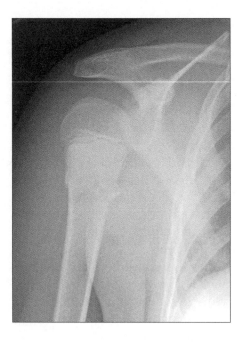

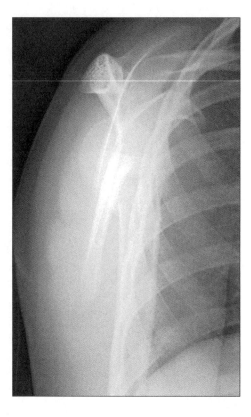

Figure 4.12 A greenstick fracture of the proximal humerus in a 13-year-old boy. Note the bulge ('torus') of cortex on the AP view (left) and the degree of angulation that is only apparent on the lateral view (right).

Figure 4.13 This is a complete fracture through the growth plate of the humeral head in a 10-year-old boy who fell from a tree. The epiphysis has slipped and rotated significantly and requires surgical intervention to reduce the fracture. There is a risk that the blood supply is compromised in this type of fracture due to the degree of displacement, but the reduction was very successful in this case.

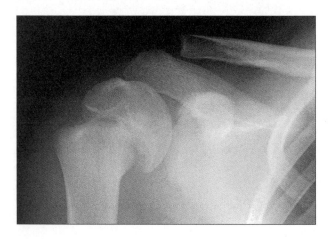

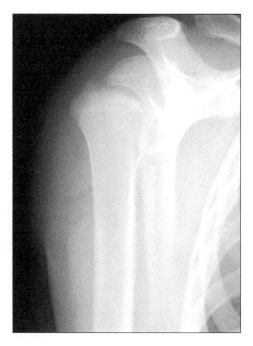

Greater tuberosity fractures

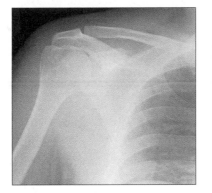

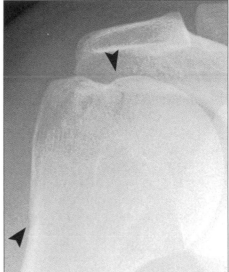

Figure 4.14 There is a fracture of the greater tuberosity (see black arrowheads on detail view). These are commonly missed and can be very subtle. Scrutinize the entire cortex of the humeral head looking for breaks or steps.

These can be very subtle and may be seen in association with a dislocation. In avulsion fractures, the bone fragment can become lodged between the acromion and the humeral head, which may need surgery to dislodge it. Check this space thoroughly on the radiograph. Fractures to the proximal humerus can occur in a variety of combinations and patterns, and are best described according to site (e.g. anatomical neck) and number of fragments (e.g. 2 parts), together with the type of fractures (e.g. transverse).

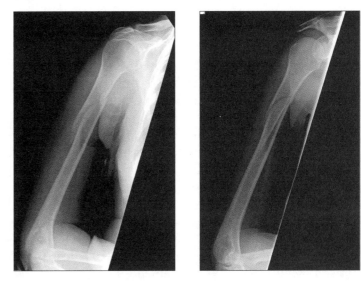

Figure 4.15 Spiral fracture of the humeral shaft. A standard AP view of the humerus was not possible because the patient was in too much pain to externally rotate the arm; the lower arm was therefore supported in a sling.

Humeral shaft fractures are usually not subtle, as shown in Figure 4.15. In this case, the fracture is spiralling around the humeral shaft. The key is to get the request right; a shoulder view may not show enough of the shaft to include the fracture. Humerus views should include shoulder and elbow joints; do not forget to check for a *fat pad sign* in the elbow (see Chapter 5 for details).

Treatment

The strong muscles usually provide good support for the humerus, and the patient is provided with a collar and cuff, giving gentle traction to the fracture. A U-slab or hanging cast is used for additional pain relief or in fractures to the shaft of the humerus. Some severe displaced fractures require manipulation, but internal fixation is reserved for fractures with four or more fragments.

Clavicular injuries

The most common mechanism of injury (94%) is as a result of a direct blow on the shoulder (McRae, 1999) followed by a fall onto the outstretched hand where the force is transmitted up the arm. The AC joint is held together by the AC ligament and the stronger coraco-clavicular ligaments (made up of the coracoid and trapezoid ligaments). Injuries to the AC joint are usually through a fall where the patient rolls onto the shoulder or a fall onto the outstretched hand (McRae, 1999), and the cervical spine should routinely be examined for bony tenderness. The severity of injury depends on the degree of ligament disruption. There may be obvious deformity and swelling over the fracture site. Patients commonly hold the arm in adduction.

Compare to the other side. Dislocation/subluxation at the sterno-clavicular joint can occur, and an obvious asymmetry at the inner (medial) end of the clavicle is noted. Check the skin colour and the patient's general appearance as sharp bone ends can perforate large vessels or lung leading to a pneumothorax. In AC-joint injuries, the outermost part of the clavicle is usually prominent, especially if all ligaments have been torn. There is localized tenderness over the site of injury, but the whole clavicle, AC-joint, shoulder and neck must be palpated to rule out associated injuries. Check the axillary nerve (over the regimental badge) and distal nerves/pulses. Active and passive movements will often be restricted due to pain. Although a standard AP view is taken, it is important to indicate that you suspect an AC-joint injury to ensure the X-ray is obtained with the patient standing and ideally both shoulders should be included in the view for comparison. Many textbooks recommend the patient has weights in each hand, to help discriminate between various grades of sprains to the ligaments. However, in the acutely injured patient, this is often too painful even with analgesia (Knapton, 1999) and often unnecessary as the treatment generally does not alter significantly.

Fractures to the clavicle are classified as medial, midshaft or lateral. Look very carefully at the entire cortex; the clavicle is S-shaped, which can prevent some fractures being clearly seen. An angled-up (15°–25°) view throws the clavicle clear of the ribs and scapula and can assist in positive fracture identification (see Figure 4.16). Fractures of the medial end of the clavicle are probably hardest to spot due to other superimposed structures on the radiograph.

Injuries to the AC joint are described according to the severity of ligament disruption and joint stability. Sprain and subluxation indicate a

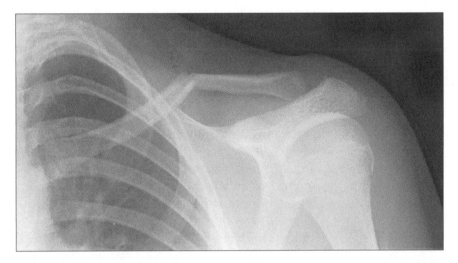

Figure 4.16 This is a typical uncomplicated fractured midshaft of clavicle, in this case in a 12-year-old boy.

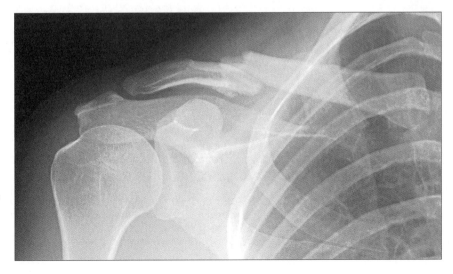

Figure 4.17 This fracture is more complicated than the previous example as there is an overriding of the ends of the fractured bone, even so the treatment is conservative.

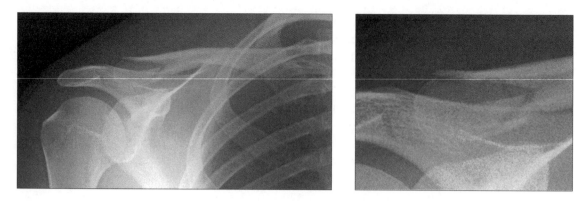

Figure 4.18 Fractures of the lateral end of the clavicle can be harder to spot – look for disruption of the AC joint. An occasionally encountered phenomenon is the absence of the extreme lateral cortex of the clavicle due to repeated trauma. This is easily confused with a more sinister lytic lesion.

tearing to the AC ligament only with the coraco-clavicular ligaments remaining intact, thus still achieving some contact between the clavicle and acromion. When reviewing a radiograph for AC-joint disruption, there are two helpful points to bear in mind. The lower cortex of the acromion and the clavicle lie on the same curved line. To assess the AC joint, trace the lower lateral border of the clavicle, which should align continuously with the lower border of the tip of the acromion. Any step in the alignment indicates subluxation, which is caused by the disruption of the coraco-clavicular and/or AC ligaments. Subluxations are graded I to III according to the degree of displacement and therefore severity of the injury. The subluxation shown in Figure 4.19b (below) is clearly a grade III, which may require surgical fixation.

More severe instability occurs when the coraco-clavicular ligaments completely tear leading to a widening gap in the coraco- clavicular space, dislocation of the AC joint and displacement of the distal clavicle. The gap between the coracoid and the clavicle is usually 1.1 to

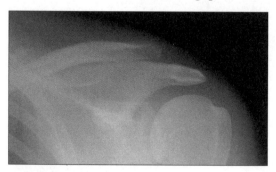
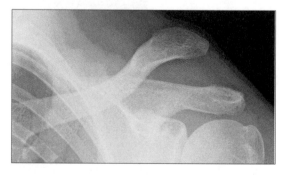

Figure 4.19 Acromio-clavicular subluxation. Trace the lower border of the clavicle, which should be continuous with the lower border of the tip of the acromion. The AC subluxations are classified according to the degree of separation vertically and the degree of widening horizontally. This grading indicates the amount of disruption of the associated ligaments. The left-hand image is of a grade I subluxation requiring only passive treatment, whereas the right-hand image is of a complete disruption requiring surgical intervention.

1.3 cm (Knapton, 1999), but a gap > 4 mm above this can indicate a partial dislocation, but a 40% or more increase in the space indicates a complete dislocation (Knapton, 1999). For a detailed description of the classification of AC disruption see Greenspan (2000).

Treatment

Most clavicular fractures are undisplaced and the treatment is purely supportive, in a broad-arm sling for approximately ten days, which can be worn underneath the clothes to provide additional support and analgesia (McRae, 1999). Although some recommend the use of a 'figure of eight' bandage, there is no evidence to support the use of this. Occasionally, attempts to correct severe displacement are made or fixed with a screw or T-plate (McRae, 1999). Dislocation of the sterno-clavicular joint is rare and should be evaluated or discussed with an orthopaedic surgeon as recurrent subluxation may occur in the future.

AC-joint treatment is usually supportive in a broad-arm sling, even when displacement is severe. Surgery is rarely performed but may be undertaken for patients involved in heavy manual labour, as complications associated with operative treatment are common.

Fractures to the scapula

These injuries indicate a high degree of mechanical force, i.e. fall from a height or a motorbike accident, and the c-spine must be examined. At times, a full trauma assessment must be undertaken. Swelling and bruising may be extensive in fractures to the neck of the scapula. There will be localized tenderness around the fracture site. The scapula serves as an attachment for several muscles, and any movements that involve the scapula will generally be restricted, owing to the patient's discomfort.

Scrutinize the AP view and trace the entire border. The fracture may be seen only on the lateral scapula view where the blade of the scapula is seen in profile and clear of the ribs. It is important to check the position of the humeral head as the gleno-humeral joint may be involved.

Treatment

Scapular fractures are usually treated conservatively, except in younger patients where there is severe displacement and damage to the glenoid, in which case surgical repair may be necessary. Early mobilization is encouraged as soon as the acuteness (pain and swelling) has settled.

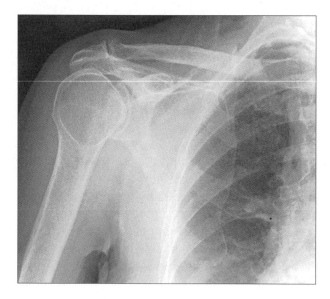

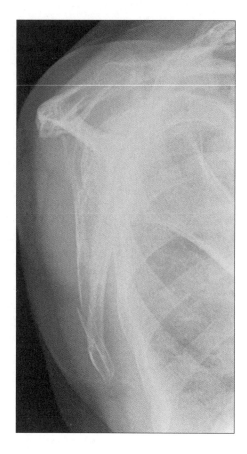

Figure 4.20 There is a fracture of the blade of the scapula near the apex. Note that this fracture cannot be reliably seen on the AP view (left) but is clearly demonstrated on the lateral view (right) where the body of the scapula is projected clear of the ribs. An axial view would not have shown the view, demonstrating the need for clear clinical information on the X-ray request form.

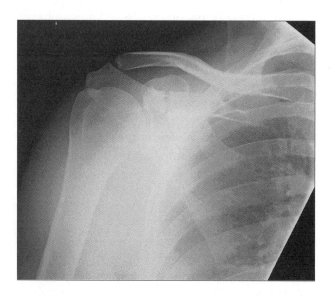

Figure 4.21 There is an unusual fracture at the base of the acromion at the point where it becomes continuous with the spine of the scapula.

Dislocations

The anterior dislocation is by far the more common and usually occurs as a result of a fall with the arm externally rotated (Dandy and Edwards, 2003). Younger patients run a risk of recurrent dislocation especially if the rehabilitation has been poor as the Glenoid Labrum may fail to reattach properly. Recurrent dislocation requires very little force. It is not uncommon for patients with a new CVA to dislocate their shoulder, but this injury is often missed. Reduction to late presentations is difficult, and need orthopaedic referral. Shoulder dislocation is extremely painful, and the patient will often hold onto the affected arm. The shoulder appears more flattened compared to the other side, with a loss of normal deltoid definition, as the head of humerus lies more medially. Start your palpation at the elbow moving along the entire shaft of the humerus and include all anatomical structures to observe for associated bony tenderness. The humeral head may be felt more anteriorly and medially or in the axilla, although this is usually too painful to palpate for. The regimental badge must be checked as shoulder dislocation carries

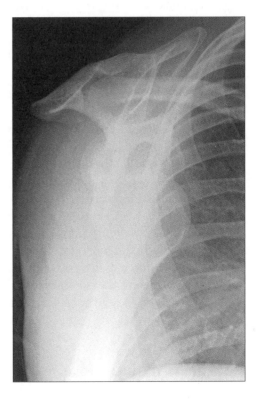
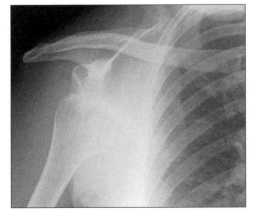

Figure 4.22 Anterior dislocation. The humeral head is inferior to the now empty glenoid and the articular surface has migrated medially. The diagnosis is confirmed on the lateral view (bottom): the humeral head is shown overlying the ribs. Note that the coracoid process always points anteriorly, which assists in orientation.

a well-known risk of axillary nerve damage. Finally, check distal nerves and pulses. The patient will resist attempts to move the shoulder.

Anterior dislocation (Figure 4.22) is obvious to spot. The humeral head is seen medial and inferior to the glenoid cavity on the AP view. An axial view will confirm the diagnosis but may be impossible due to pain in correct positioning; on the lateral scapula view the humeral head will be seen anterior to the glenoid overlying the ribs.

In cases of repeated dislocations, there may be chronic signs on the film. The Hill-Sachs lesion is a notch on the posterior aspect of the articular surface of the humeral head caused by contact with the rim of the glenoid. Bankhart's lesion is the equivalent erosion of the glenoid rim.

Treatment

If there is an associated fracture present, orthopaedics should be consulted prior to any reduction. There are several methods described to reduce a shoulder, but the key to them all is to overcome muscle spasm, which may include the use of IV opioid. The use of sedatives (e.g. Midazolam) may be required to fully overcome muscle spasm, but great care must be taken and full resuscitation equipment must be available, especially if the patient has already received opioids. General anaesthetic is reserved for failed attempts, e.g. where the humeral head has 'button holed' through the subscapularis (open reduction is then required) or where muscle spasm cannot be overcome. It is not the purpose of this book to describe common reduction techniques, as these are available in most standard orthopaedic textbooks. However, we have included one method (the hanging-arm method) that is very useful for the MIU where sedation may not be feasible.

The patient is placed lying face down on a trolley, with the affected arm hanging freely. A sandbag or bag of IV fluid can be placed under the clavicle. The weight of the hanging arm will provide gentle gravitational traction, but adequate analgesia must be given. Additional patient-administered Entonox is also useful, but nothing can replace communicating with the patient to provide distraction and relaxation.

Post-reduction radiographs are always obtained.

Posterior dislocations

Posterior dislocations (Figure 4.23) are more subtle radiologically – two views are required to absolutely exclude a posterior dislocation; however, most are apparent on the AP film. When the joint is not dislocated, there is normally a 'crescent sign' (see Figure 4.4). This occurs because the articular surface of the humeral head is superimposed over the glenoid producing an overlapping of the structures. The absence of this sign is suggestive of posterior dislocation. In addition, the normal asymmetric appearance of the humeral head is lost and appears more like a light bulb. In both cases, a second view is required for confirmation.

Treatment

Reduction is advised, but this is unstable and the patient should be referred to the orthopaedic surgeons.

Non-trauma

Patients presenting with a painful shoulder but no clear history of trauma should have a very detailed history obtained, as many life-threatening problems manifest themselves with pain in the shoulder (Wardrope and English, 1998; Purcell, 2003):

- spine pathology
- ectopic pregnancy
- myocardial infarction
- lung pathology (e.g. pneumonia, pneumothorax or tumours)

The history must include PMH, onset and duration of problem, type of pain, associated symptoms and any aggravating/relieving factors. If you cannot find any local/specific shoulder pathology, you must have a high index of suspicion for referred pain. X-rays may be indicated even

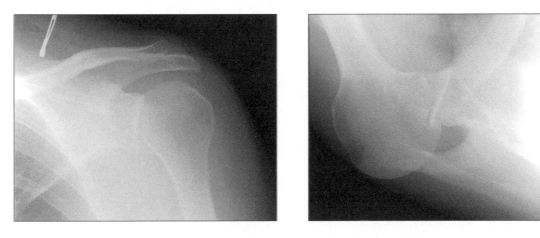

Figure 4.23 Posterior dislocation. Look carefully at the AP view (left) of the joint; there is an absence of congruency in the joint and the crescent sign is absent. In addition, the humeral head appears more symmetrical – the light bulb sign. The axial view (right) confirms that the humeral head is posterior to the glenoid. Note also that the glenoid has notched into the articular surface of the humerus.

if there is no clear history of trauma but the patient presents with localized bony tenderness – especially in the elderly or patients with a history of carcinoma. The clinical examination follows the same principles as for traumatic injuries, although in more detail. Examine joints above and below and the whole spine. Remember that referred pain may not follow dermatome pattern (Wardrope and English, 1998). Observe the general state of the patient – is there evidence of systemic disease (e.g. clubbing, infection or anaemia)? Note the respiration rate, pattern and depth. Note any swelling, deformity or discoloration. Check the skin temperature. Is it hot, cold or clammy? Obtain vital signs, including temperature, then palpate to identify any areas of tenderness noticing both soft tissue and bone. Include a full neurovascular assessment.

It is outside the scope of this book to discuss every non-traumatic condition affecting the shoulder, as most non-traumatic shoulder complaints do not require an X-ray. One of the exceptions is the calcification of supraspinatus tendon.

Calcific supraspinatus tendinitis

The cause of this is uncertain, but calcium salts are deposited in the tendon. A typical history is in patients aged 30–45 who suddenly develop an acute onset of pain that increases over 24–48 hours to become agonizing. It is not related to any activity/movement. There is no clear history of injury or over-use. Calcific supraspinatus tendonitis differentiates from adhesive capsulitis ('frozen shoulder'), which has a gradual onset of pain. X-ray (Figure 4.24) will show calcification within the supraspinatus tendon.

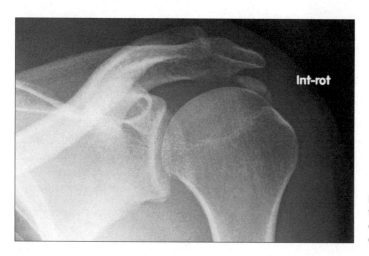

Figure 4.24 Calcification is seen within the supraspinatus tendon. This is often a cause of pain and indicative of rotator cuff disease.

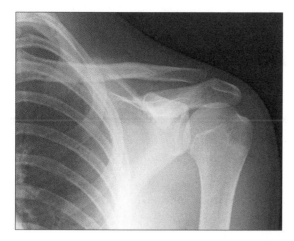

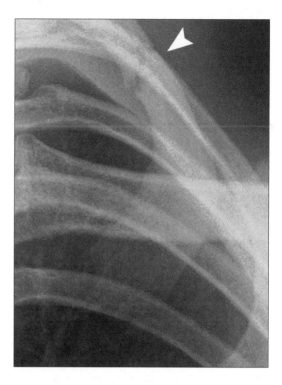

Figure 4.25 This is a rare finding, but the abnormality must be detected. There is a fracture of the first rib in this young adult caused by a fall from a horse. It is easily missed (see arrowhead on detail view) simply because the focus of concentration by the observer will naturally be on the bony anatomy of the shoulder rather than the ribs.

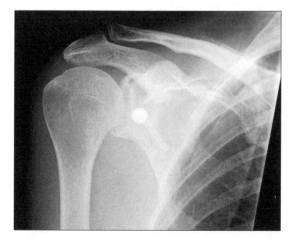

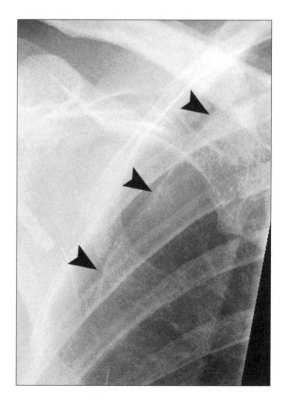

Figure 4.26 There is no acute bone abnormality seen in this image, but you need to look carefully at the edge of the lung fields. There is a small pneumothorax, which is demonstrated as a dense line just inside the lateral wall of the chest – see arrowheads on detail view (right). There are no lung markings (lung vessels) beyond this line, which represents the edge of the collapsed lung. This case clearly needs a decision as to whether aspiration or a chest drain is required, and an experienced opinion is required.

Chapter 5

The distal humerus and elbow

Review of core anatomy

The elbow consists of three joints all contained in a synovial capsule: the radio-humeral and the ulnar-humeral joints form a hinged joint with uniaxial movements. The proximal radio-ulnar joint is included as part of the elbow joint, as it is responsible for rotational movements.

The distal end of the humerus consists of two cartilage-covered structures: the rounded capitellum (capitulum in some textbooks), which articulates with the radial head, and a flatter grooved part known as the trochlea, which articulates with the proximal ulna. There are two 'hollows' located in the distal humerus. One just above the capitellum known as the radial fossa and another, coranoid fossa, just above the trochlea (see Figure 5.1).

On the anterior surface, the shaft of the humerus broadens distally into a triangular shape with two bony prominences called the medial and lateral epicondyles, with the medial epicondyle being the more prominent (Purcell, 2003; Dean and Pegington, 1996) – see Figure 5.1.

The forearm is made up of two long bones: the radius and ulna, which are discussed in further detail in Chapter 6. The proximal end of the radius terminates in a round head sitting on a restricted neck.

During flexion, the radial head fits into the radial fossa. The proximal end of the ulna expands and deepens into a groove, with a projection anteriorly called the coranoid process and a posterior process known as the olecranon (see Figure 5.1). During flexion, the trochlea is grasped at the front by the coranoid process, which fits into the coranoid fossa and posteriorly by the olecranon, which fits into the olecranon fossa during extension. On the lateral aspect of the coranoid process, a small hollow (radial notch) is found which enables rotation of the radial head.

The proximal radio-ulnar joint is held together by a strong ligament (the annular ligament) around the head of the radius and the radial notch (Dean and Pegington, 1996), keeping the radial head close to the ulna while allowing it to rotate. The elbow is supported by the strong radial and ulnar collateral ligaments, which limit adduction

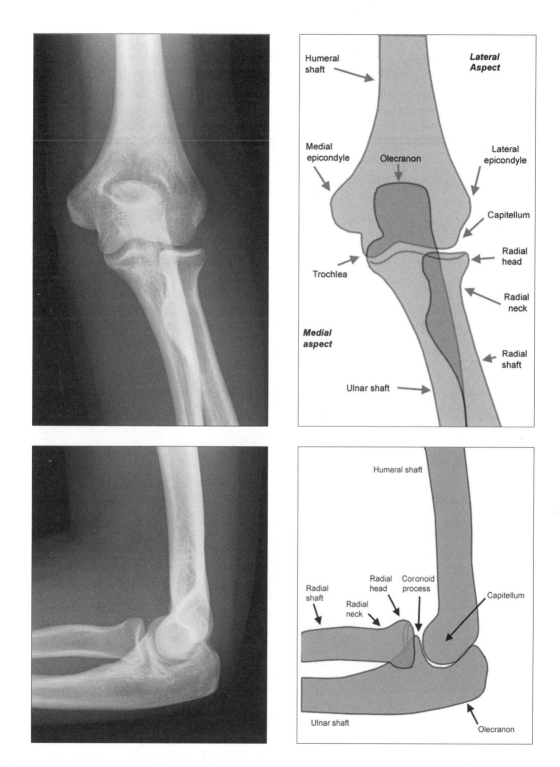

Figure 5.1 Normal adult elbow views AP (top) and lateral (bottom) together with schematic diagrams of the essential anatomical features visible on the radiographs.

and abduction. The radial collateral ligament arises from the lateral epicondyle and inserts into the annular ligament on the radial notch. The ulnar collateral ligament arises from the medial epicondyle and spreads out in a fan-like pattern to the coranoid process anteriorly and the olecranon posteriorly.

The capsule is lined with a synovial membrane, and in between this membrane and the capsule are fat pads that act as cushions to absorb forces across the joint. An awareness of these fat pads is important in radiographic interpretation.

Standard projections

AP
lateral

Additional projections

radial head view

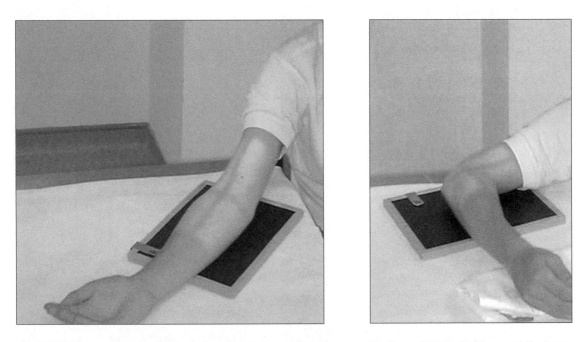

Figure 5.2 X-ray positioning. The technique for obtaining elbow views requires the patient to sit sideways at the X-ray table and supinate the extended arm to give the AP view (left). This is particularly painful if the patient has a radial head or neck fracture as the radial head is forced to rotate within the annular ligament. Compromise views are sometimes taken if the patient cannot tolerate full extension, with the elbow only partially extended, although this will always give rise to some degree of distortion. The lateral view (right) is obtained by raising the X-ray table and flexing the elbow to 90° with the wrist supported on a small pad. To achieve the additional radial head view, the patient is positioned as for the lateral but the X-ray beam is angled at about 40° up the humerus.

AP view

The patient sits sideways at the X-ray table with the arm extended and the hand palm uppermost. Note that it can be extremely painful for the patient to adopt this position in the presence of the injury or fracture. The distal third of the humerus and the proximal third of the radius and ulna should be demonstrated on the film.

When scrutinizing the radiographs, note that on the AP view many of the bony structures are superimposed; however, the joint spaces should appear congruent and the radial head should align with the capitellum. Pay particular attention to the radial head and the radial neck; fractures in these regions can be very subtle.

A familiarity with the normal alignments of the elbow joint is absolutely crucial in spotting subtle abnormalities. Look at the AP view (Figure 5.3, left). A line drawn through the centre of the proximal radial shaft and neck should pass through the capitellum. On the lateral view, this alignment should be maintained; any misalignment is indicative of radial dislocation. This rule holds true even when the

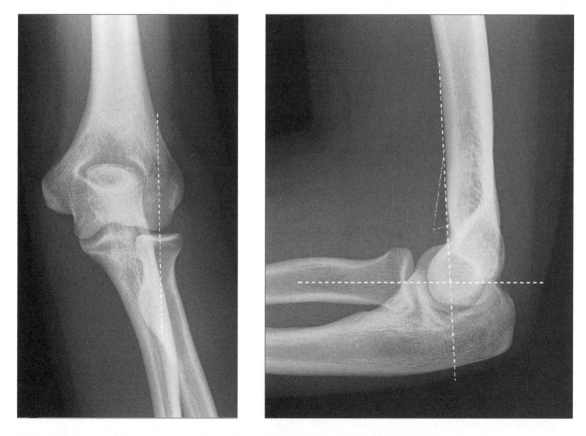

Figure 5.3 Normal alignments in the elbow joint (left) and normal anterior fat pad (right).

projections are not truly AP or lateral as the radial head is a circular structure held in position within the circular annular ligament.

To check for subtle supracondylar fracture look at the anterior humeral line. This is a line drawn on the lateral view along the anterior border of the humerus (see Figure 5.3, right). Approximately one-third of the capitellum should be seen lying anterior to this line. If the amount of capitellum seen is less than one-third, a supracondylar fracture should be suspected and the humeral cortex scrutinized for a fracture.

The elbow joint, as with all synovial joints, is encapsulated by a synovial membrane containing fluid secreted by the membrane. In the presence of trauma, the amount of fluid within the capsule increases. This pushes out fat pads lying anteriorly and posteriorly in the distal humerus. There is normally a portion of anterior fat pad always visible on the lateral view as a slightly darker triangle seen just above the capitellum on the anterior humeral line – fat being of lower density than the surrounding soft tissues and therefore absorbing fewer X-rays. The normal anterior fat pad forms an angle of about 20° with the anterior cortex of the humerus. If the elbow suffers traumatic injury, the resultant effusion forces out the fat pad such that the anterior fat pad angle increases and the posterior fat pad is then rendered visible against the posterior humeral cortex (Figure 5.4). Note that the posterior fat pad is normally completely contained within a bony cavity and therefore not seen on the normal uninjured elbow's lateral view.

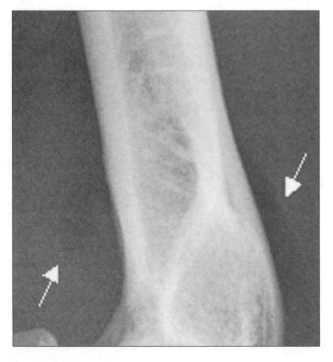

Figure 5.4 Anterior and posterior fat pads rendered visible by a joint effusion (white arrows).

Elbow injuries and fractures

Clinical examination

Most injuries to the elbow occur as a result of indirect trauma, e.g. a fall onto the outstretched hand, which is also the common mechanism of injury for many shoulder and wrist injuries, and the whole of the limb must always be examined (Wardrope and English, 1998). Start at the shoulder and cover the whole of the humerus. The radius and ulna are bound firmly together both proximally and distally through several ligaments. The net effect is that of a bundle of sticks tied together in a parallelogram acting as one (McRae, 1999). Therefore, there is a high likelihood of injuries to both bones, except when direct trauma has occurred. The onus is on the clinician positively to exclude injury to the other bones, and a thorough clinical examination of the wrist must be undertaken. Any positive findings must be stated on the X-ray request to ensure both joints are included, if so indicated.

The brachial artery runs down through the medial aspect of the upper arm and divides into the radial and ulnar arteries after crossing the cubital region. The ulnar, median and radial nerves and the brachial artery all pass through the elbow, and damage to these structures is a well-documented complication of elbow injuries. Consequently, a full neurovascular assessment of the whole limb must be undertaken.

Look

When the forearm is in its anatomical position (i.e. the forearm is fully extended, supinated and the palm of the hand is facing forward), the upper arm and forearm are not in the same line. Rather the forearm is directed in a 10°–15° valgus angle (larger for women) known as the *carrying angle* (Purcell, 2003). The purpose of this angle is to clear the extended forearm off the side of the hips when swinging the arms during walking, especially when carrying heavy loads. Old injuries, especially supracondylar fractures, may alter this angle and are most noticeable when compared with the opposite side (McRae, 1999).

Observe how the patient is holding the arm. Patients with injuries to the elbow often hold the arm in some degree of flexion with the forearm mid-rotated. Note any obvious deformity – there are a few conditions that will cause an obvious deformity to the elbow: supracondylar fractures, dislocation of the elbow and dislocation of the radial head, with or without an associated ulnar fracture. Is there any bruising? This can take a few days to appear but may then be extensive, with a gravitational spread to the wrist. Note any swelling. Is it localized, as in olecranon bursitis, or more generalized, as in effusion?

Feel

Palpate all bony landmarks to identify the point of maximum tenderness, starting at the shoulder including the epicondyles, olecranon, radial head, shaft of radius/ulna and finally the wrist.

Move

The elbow joint is in 0° extension when the arm is in its anatomical position, although 10°–15° hyperextension is common. Loss of full extension is a good indication of injury, and is best noticed when compared with the opposite limb. Flexion is approximately 150°, but may vary depending on the patient's musculature. At the proximal radio-ulnar joint, pronation and supination occurs. The elbow should be isolated by holding the upper arm close to the body, as the shoulder joint can also initiate these movements.

Several muscles are involved in the movement of the elbow, with the main contributors as follows:

- biceps: flexes the forearm when the arm is supinated
- brachioradialis and brachial: flex the elbow in either supination or pronation
- triceps: extends the elbow
- supinator: supination
- pronator teres and pronator quadratus: pronation

Any rupturing of the triceps can lead to avulsion fractures. It is important to distinguish these injuries from closed rupture of the biceps tendon, as avulsion fractures may need surgical repair. Check active and passive movements of both elbows, but only undertake resisted movements if you don't suspect fractures or dislocations.

Radial head/neck and capitellum fractures

The mechanism of injury is usually as a result of a fall onto an outstretched hand, where the energy is transmitted up the radius and the radial head hits the capitellum, which may additionally fracture. It is essential to examine the whole limb. The patient usually holds the limb in some degree of flexion. Swelling and bruising may not be apparent initially. Local tenderness of the radial head can be difficult to ascertain through the thick forearm muscles, but becomes more apparent when the head is rotated under pressure. Place your thumb in the space laterally between the radial head and humerus and gently supinate and pronate the elbow while you continue to palpate

(McRae, 1999). Finally, check distal nerves and vessels. There is usually a loss of full extension, while pronation/supination is often intact but painful. A loss of extension together with a clear history should lead you to suspect a radial head fracture and your X-ray request form should indicate this, to ensure you get the best views possible.

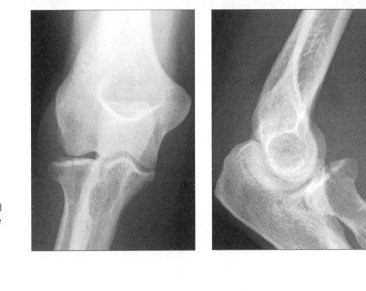

Figure 5.5 This is a classic radial head fracture with some fracture displacement. Note the anterior and posterior fat pads are clearly visible on the lateral view (right) indicating a significant joint effusion.

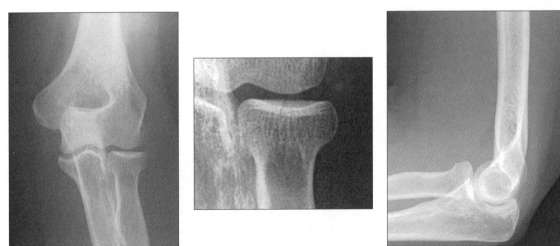

Figure 5.6 Another classic radial head fracture commonly presenting as an acute injury. In this case, the fracture appearance is much more subtle than in Figure 5.5; however, the positive fat pad sign in the lateral view (right) gives a clue as to the severity of the injury and raises the possibility of a fracture being present. The fracture is perceptible in the AP view (left and centre) but could be missed, particularly if the images are taken soon after injury. Note that it cannot be reliably detected on the lateral view of the radial head itself (right). A radial head view may be done to confirm the diagnosis; however, this is unlikely to change the management in view of the clinical signs and the positive joint effusion.

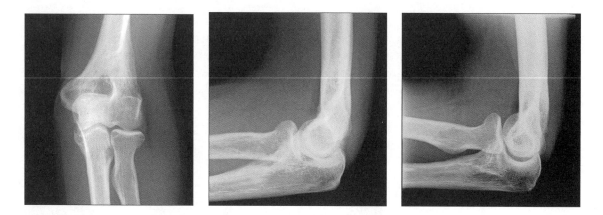

Figure 5.7 There is a very subtle radial head fracture demonstrated by this examination. Unusually, there is no joint effusion; this can happen if the injury occurs a number of days before the images are taken. The right-hand radiograph is the additional angled view, which throws the radial head clear of the ulna and can often demonstrate a radial head fracture not apparent on the standard views.

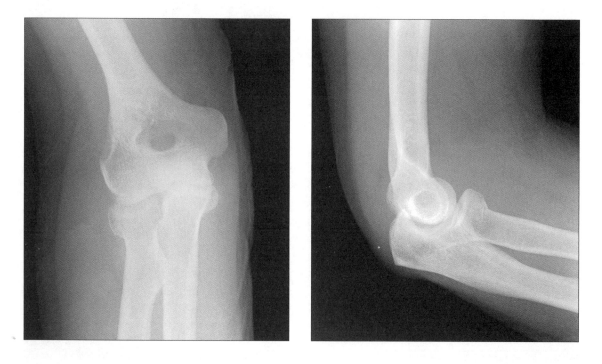

Figure 5.8 This examination demonstrates a radial head fracture and also an example of a normal variant. The olecranon fossa in this patient completely penetrates the humerus and is thus an olecranon foramen. Note the prominent joint effusion associated with the fracture on the lateral view (right).

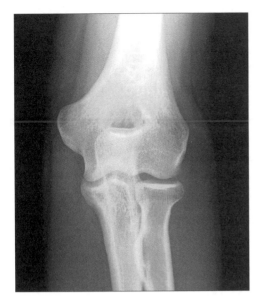 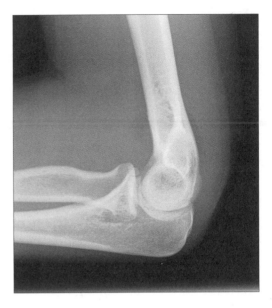

Figure 5.9 This is an uncommon, and possibly missable, undisplaced fracture of the coranoid process of the ulna. Because the coranoid process is superimposed over the radial head on the lateral view (right), the break in the cortex does not stand out clearly. On the AP view (left), the fracture is shown *en face* and is completely invisible. The associated joint effusion is clearly seen. This type of fracture emphasizes the need for a systematic scrutiny of the film: trace the cortex of all three bones and check the alignments and the soft-tissue signs.

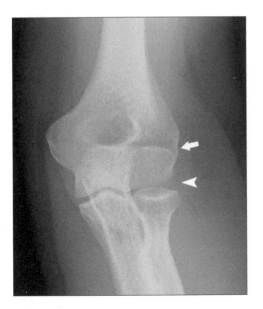 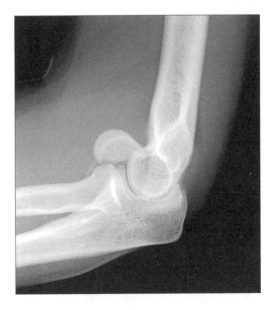

Figure 5.10 In this image, the capitellum has been avulsed anteriorly. This comminuted fracture is clearly demonstrated on the lateral view (right), but on the AP view (left) it is shown by the sclerotic line overlying the distal humerus (white arrow) and by the irregularity of the cortex where the capitellum would normally lie (white arrowhead). Note the joint effusion.

Treatment

If a flake fracture to the capitellum is seen, refer the patient to orthopaedics as the patient may need loose body excised. Other capitellum fractures can be treated in a sling and followed up by orthopaedic surgeons, as they are at risk of developing osteoarthritis and osteochondritis dissicans.

Radial head/neck fractures account for about 50% of elbow fractures (Nicholson and Driscoll, 1993) and are treated according to severity, but always be aware of any evidence of loose bodies in the joint space (McRae, 1999):

- Undisplaced/minimal displaced fractures are treated in a broad-arm sling, and analgesia and early (after two to three weeks) mobilization. Some radial head fractures are not always visible on initial X-ray. Even in the absence of raised fat pads, clinically suspected radial head fractures without radiological evidence should be treated as a fracture.
- Displaced fractures with > 30° angulation should be referred for possible open reduction and internal fixation, although at times the fracture is treated conservatively for a few months and then, depending on the severity of restricted movements, late excision of the radial head is performed.
- Grossly comminuted fractures are treated by immediate excision of the radial head.

Myositis ossificans

Myositis ossificans is callus formation in the tissue near a joint, and is a well-documented complication in elbow injuries causing a severe restriction of movement. It follows a too-early or a too-aggressive mobilization or after passive extension of the elbow joint (McRae, 1999). Early removal of the callus is counter-productive, as it usually leads to massive recurrence. Late excision (six to twelve months) is the treatment of choice (McRae, 1999).

Monteggia's fracture

One complicated elbow injury involving the radial head is the so-called Monteggia's fracture (Figure 5.12) where there is a fracture of the proximal ulna and dislocation of the radial head. Occasionally, the

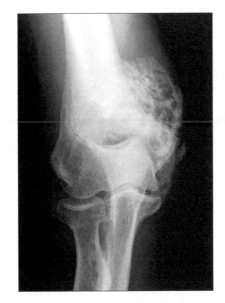

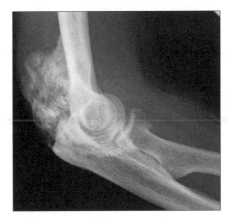

Figure 5.11 Myositis ossificans. Note the excessive callus formation in the soft tissues.

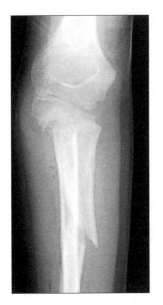

Figure 5.12 Monteggia's fracture dislocation of the forearm. The comminuted ulnar fracture in this 9-year-old boy who fell off his bike is obvious, but perhaps the radial head dislocation is not as simple to detect. Always follow the rules of alignment and it will be seen that the radial shaft does not intersect the capitellum on the lateral view (right). Note the presence of air in the soft tissues, indicating a compound fracture.

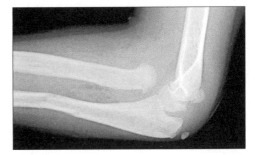

ulnar fracture may be so proximal that it is mistaken for an olecranon fracture. The fracture is very obvious and the dislocation of the radial head easily missed, unless you actively look for it. You should never diagnose an isolated dislocated radial head or single shaft of ulnar fracture until you have positively ruled out a Monteggia's fracture. This fracture needs immediate referral to orthopaedics.

Olecranon fractures

Approximately one-third of elbow fractures are to the olecranon (Nicholson and Driscoll, 1993). The mechanism of injury is usually as a result of a direct fall onto the flexed elbow, where the distal humerus acts like a chisel splitting the olecranon (Dandy and Edwards, 2003) but can occur as a result of a fall onto the outstretched hand with the elbow flexed. In addition, avulsion fractures of the olecranon, which are caused by a rupture of the triceps tendons at their insertion, also occur. There is usually significant swelling and the elbow is held in flexion, and significant localized tenderness is found. Ensure you palpate both shoulder and wrist. Full neurovascular assessment is required. There is a loss of extension and the patient will resist all attempts to move the elbow.

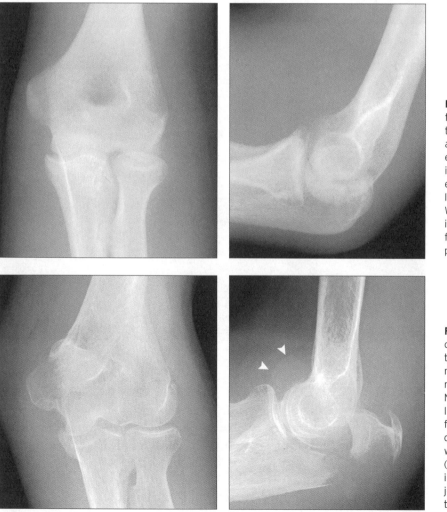

Figure 5.13 There is a fracture of the tip of the olecranon with an associated joint effusion. The fracture is undisplaced but only easily seen on the lateral view (right). Without immobilization, this fracture would probably displace.

Figure 5.14 This is a displaced fracture of the olecranon that requires surgical reduction and fixation. Note also the tug lesion at the tip of the fragment, which is degenerative. The white arrowheads (lateral view, right) indicate the enormous joint effusion seen in the soft tissues.

Treatment

Olecranon fractures are usually displaced and need referral for internal fixation. Undisplaced, hairline fractures can be treated in an above-elbow plaster cast.

Dislocated elbow

The mechanism of injury is a fall onto the outstretched hand with the elbow in near full extension. The ulna usually dislocates posterior-laterally, and may be accompanied by fractures to the coranoid process, medial epicondyle or radial head/neck. There is obvious deformity and swelling. It is extremely painful and the patient will guard it and resist any attempts to move the joint. Again, check the distal neurovascular function, as there is a high risk of neurovascular compromise.

Figure 5.15 Elbow dislocation. There is a total dislocation of the elbow joint with loss of normal alignment. Follow the rules of alignment and it will be seen that the shaft of the radius does not intersect the capitellum on the AP view (left) or on the lateral view (right).

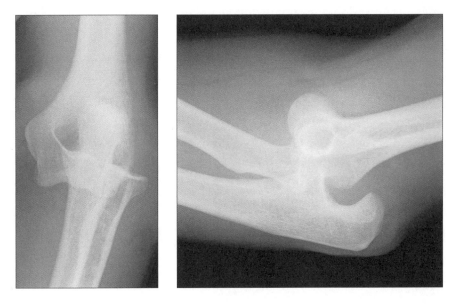

Treatment

The treatment is reduction. A post-reduction X-ray must be taken. If there are no associated fractures, the elbow is immobilized in a sling for two weeks to encourage early mobilization. Associated fractures are treated accordingly.

Paediatric elbow examinations

The paediatric elbow probably causes more anxiety than any other plain film extremity examinations. This is, in part, due to the complexity and distribution of the ossification centres and the potential for mistaking normal appearances for a fracture and dismissing pathology as a normal appearance. In addition, good projections in an injured and frightened child are often difficult to obtain, and the radiographer needs to apply a sympathetic modification to their radiographic technique in order to obtain adequate diagnostic images. In the adult elbow, the radial head is the most common element to fracture, whereas this is rarely seen in children. Thus, it is important to appreciate that although the principles of examination of the elbow radiographs are the same the resultant abnormalities may be quite different.

Figure 5.16 illustrates the normal appearance of the elbow in a 14-year-old boy. The ossification process commences as a dot of bony material at the centre of the cartilage 'model' that progressively enlarges and adopts the final adult shape by fusing with the main bone shaft. Thus, the capitellum in a baby appears oval but in an 8-year-old

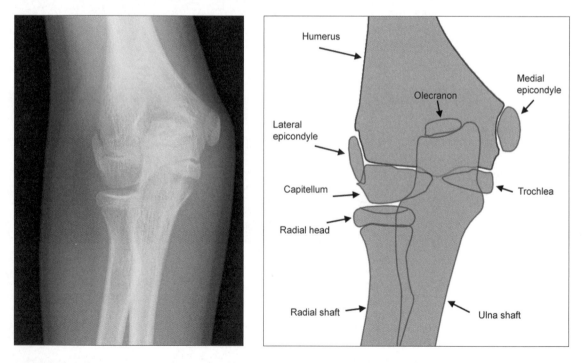

Figure 5.16 AP radiograph of a normal elbow of a 14-year-old boy showing all secondary ossification centres present and a schematic diagram of the same image. Note that the age of appearance and subsequent fusion of the ossification centres with the main bone shaft is variable from individual to individual.

is a more complex shape as the cartilage margin becomes mineralized (see Figure 5.17). During development, they are seen on the radiographs as separate entities but are distinguishable from avulsion fractures as they are normally smooth and rounded. Even when they are irregular or fragmented, they occupy expected locations, which is why being familiar with the normal appearance is so important. Occasionally, these separate ossification centres persist into adulthood

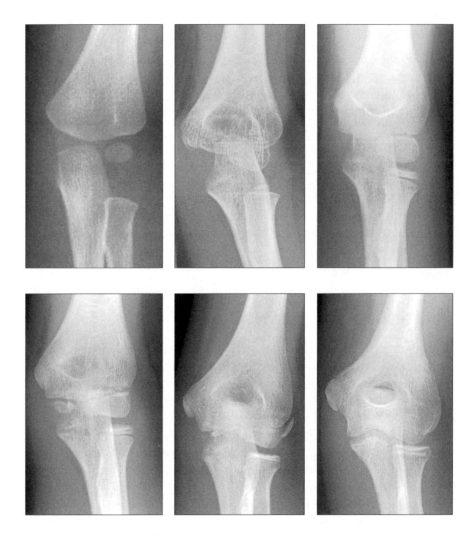

Figure 5.17 Ossification centres in the paediatric elbow at ages: 11m, 3y, 6y, 9y, 12y, 15y. In the top left image, only the capitellum is visible but is only partially mineralized; in the top right image, the radial head and internal (medial) epicondyle are now also visible and the capitellum has achieved a more adult form; in the centre left image the radial head has expanded and the trochlea is now just visible; in the centre right image these ossification centres are more fully formed and the olecranon is just visible; in the bottom left image the lateral epicondyle is now visible, and in the bottom right image the ossification centres are now almost completely fused. Note that the order of ossification follows the CRITOL order (see text above), which is invariable.

and can mimic a fracture. The mnemonic 'CRITOL' is useful in helping to memorize these ossification centres and the strict order in which they ossify:

Capitellum   articulates with the radial head
Radial head
Internal epicondyle   strictly the medial epicondyle
Trochlea   articulates with the coranoid process of the ulna
Olecranon
Lateral epicondyle

Note: the capitellum, radial head and trochlea are *epiphyses* as they form part of a joint surface, whereas the medial and lateral epicondyles and the olecranon are *apophyses* as they are sites of tendon or ligament attachment but do not articulate with another bone, nor do they contribute to increasing bone length.

The sequence of images in Figure 5.17 shows the development of the elbow up to the age of 12. The different anatomical elements of the elbow are all actually present at birth and exist not as bone but as radiolucent cartilage. Subsequently, they ossify – become mineralized and therefore visible on the radiograph – as the child grows. Note that the shape as well as the size of the ossification centres change, as mineralization progresses.

Paediatric elbow injuries

There are a great variety of potential injuries to the paediatric elbow; however, in a text of this nature it is necessary to limit those described to the most commonly encountered. For a fuller, very readable account see Thornton and Gyll (1999).

The most common paediatric elbow injury is the supracondylar fracture with a peak incidence at 4–8 years (Thornton and Gyll, 1999). When the fracture is complete, there is a risk of damage to the brachial artery or medial and ulnar nerves, and great caution should be exercised when positioning for X-ray. Essentially, the elbow should be X-rayed with the arm in the presenting positioning with appropriate modification of technique, i.e. horizontal beam as necessary. In the patient who presents with severe pain and obvious deformity, one view in order to demonstrate the fracture is sufficient with further views or fluoroscopic screening under GA. It is a mistake for the radiographer to persist in trying to obtain two textbook views, as this will result in unnecessary pain and potentially increase the extent of the injury.

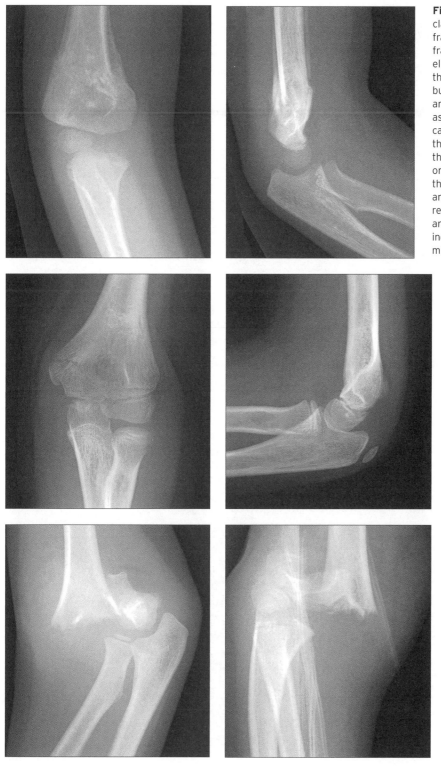

Figure 5.18 This is a classic supracondylar fracture, the most common fracture of the paediatric elbow. On the AP view (left) the fracture line is visible but the degree of angulation cannot be assessed from this view and can belie the seriousness of the injury. Look carefully at the anterior humeral line on the lateral view (right): the distal humerus is angulated posteriorly resulting in none showing anterior to this line indicating that a fracture must be present.

Figure 5.19 This would probably be more correctly described as an intracondylar rather than a supracondylar fracture. Note that there is no fracture displacement and thus there is no misalignment seen on the lateral view (right), although there is a prominent associated joint effusion.

Figure 5.20 Grossly displaced and comminuted supracondylar fracture. Note the degree of fracture displacement. This injury requires very careful handling and the absolute minimum possible manipulation by the radiographer in order to achieve a view of the joint to allow referral. Any further examination of the injury can be carried out under GA using fluoroscopy.

Figure 5.21 This injury has resulted in the detachment of the capitellum together with a large fragment of the lateral humeral metaphysis (condyle). The radial head remains in articulation with the capitellum. A posterior fat pad is visible, but it is not a true lateral view (right) and the signs of an effusion are less reliable. This type of fracture is relatively common at any age.

Figure 5.22 Fracture of the lateral condyle of the distal humerus in a 15-year-old boy. Note the fracture line communicates with the joint in the region of the capitellum. The medial and lateral epicondyles are still partially unfused.

Figure 5.23 Avulsion and displacement of the medial epicondyle apophysis. This injury demonstrates the requirement for a knowledge of the site and order of the ossification centres (CRITOL, see above). The AP view (left) shows the medial epicondyle displaced inferiorly to the level of the radial head (arrowhead), and on the lateral view (right) it is seen superimposed over the capitellum in line with the centre of the radial head (arrow). On the lateral view, the olecranon ossification centre is just visible (arrowhead) but the lateral epicondyle is not yet mineralized.

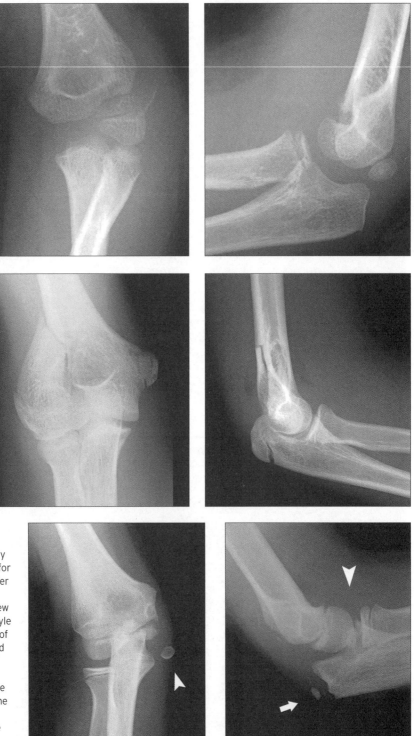

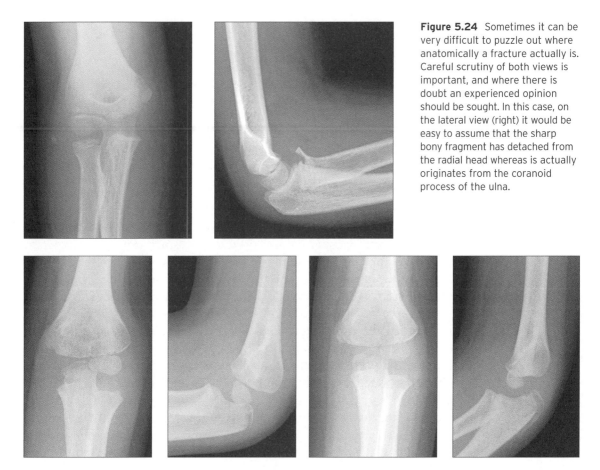

Figure 5.24 Sometimes it can be very difficult to puzzle out where anatomically a fracture actually is. Careful scrutiny of both views is important, and where there is doubt an experienced opinion should be sought. In this case, on the lateral view (right) it would be easy to assume that the sharp bony fragment has detached from the radial head whereas is actually originates from the coranoid process of the ulna.

Figure 5.25 These four views are of the same elbow. The left pair are within twelve hours post-injury. The images appear unremarkable; however, the positioning of the lateral view (second left) is poor due to the child being in severe pain. The patient was X-rayed again two weeks later, and there is periosteal reaction seen around the cortex of the olecranon. In fact, what was thought to be the olecranon ossification centre in the initial lateral view (second left) is a fracture. In retrospect, following the CRITOL sequence of ossification, the capitellum, radial head and internal (medial) epicondyle are visible but the trochlea is not; the olecranon should, therefore, also not be visible.

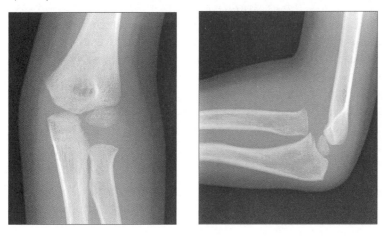

Figure 5.26 Look carefully at both of the views. No fracture is visible because there isn't one. In fact, the AP view (left) is completely normal; however, an examination of the bony alignments on the lateral view (right) reveals that the radial head is dislocated anteriorly from its normal articulation with the capitellum. This is an uncommon injury that must be reduced under GA. Note the joint effusion indicating trauma to the joint.

Chapter 6
The forearm and wrist

Review of core anatomy

The forearm is made up of two long bones: on the lateral side ('thumb' side might be easier to remember) the radius, and on the medial side the ulna. The radius at the elbow joint is shaped in a round head (see Chapter 5) and becomes wider and thicker distally. The ulna is wide at the elbow forming the olecranon but narrows considerably distally at the wrist. Both the radius and the ulna can be felt on the dorsal aspect of the wrist as two bony prominences called the styloid processes, which serve as attachments for ligaments (Dean and Pegington, 1996). In between the radius and ulna lies the interosseous membrane from where many muscles originate. Although the radius and ulna are separate and only held together with ligaments, in terms of function they operate as one, which is an important concept to bear in mind when assessing patients following trauma. The distal ulna articulates with the radius at the distal radio-ulnar joint held together by the triangular cartilage. This cartilage is attached to the distal end of the radius and the ulnar styloid. Fractures to the distal radius or ulna often result in disruption and instability to this joint and may lead to an associated avulsion fracture of the ulnar styloid.

The actual wrist consists of eight carpal bones lying in two rows forming several highly mobile joints held tightly together by several strong ligaments preventing excessive movements. The proximal row contains the scaphoid, lunate, triquetral and pisiform and the distal row the trapezium, trapezoid, capitate and hamate (see Figure 6.6, right). The scaphoid is the largest of the carpal bones and bridges the two rows making this bone vulnerable to damage from hyperextension injury, as its waist is over-stressed. The distal radius articulates with the proximal carpal bones at the radio-carpal joint. The distal row of carpal bones articulates with the bones of the hand at the carpo-metacarpal joint.

Clinical examination

Most injuries to the wrist occur as a result of indirect trauma, e.g. a fall onto the outstretched hand, which is also the common mechanism of injury for many shoulder and elbow injuries. Consequently, the whole of the limb must always be examined. The radius and ulna are bound together both proximally and distally through several ligaments. The net effect is that of a bundle of sticks tied together in a parallelogram acting as one (McRae, 1999). Therefore, there is high likelihood of injuries to both bones, except when direct trauma has occurred. The onus is on the clinician positively to exclude injury to the other bone, and a thorough clinical examination of the whole forearm and the elbow must be undertaken. Any positive findings must be stated on the X-ray request to ensure both joints are included, if so indicated.

It is essential to ascertain and document the patient's hand dominance and occupation/hobbies, as some injuries may severely affect the patient's livelihood or the treatment may alter depending on the degree of function required in the patient's daily living. Be careful not to underestimate the severity of soft-tissue injuries, as some can be as disabling as fractures. The term 'sprain' is a common diagnosis, but is very unspecific (Wardrope and English, 1998). The 'sprained wrist' is the second-most-common diagnostic error made in the A&E department, and up to 2% of patients with this diagnosis have a more significant injury that was missed (Guly, 2002).

The forearm and wrist obtain their vascular supply from the brachial artery, which divides into the radial and ulnar arteries at the cubital fossa at the elbow. The radial artery crosses the anatomical snuff box before dividing to supply the hand and fingers. The ulnar artery follows the ulnar nerve through the wrist before dividing to supply the ulnar aspect of the hand. The arteries subdivide into several branches, some of which anatomizes to form an arch. This collateral circulation ensures that when one artery has been divided (e.g. from trauma) the circulation is not impaired (Dandy and Edwards, 2003). Each finger receives a palmer digital artery to each side of the finger running alongside the digital nerve.

Motor and sensory nervous supply are via the median, ulnar and radial nerves and are assessed distally in the fingers, which is discussed in detail in Chapter 7. However, the importance of ensuring this is carried out and documented cannot be over-emphasized.

Look

Some wrist injuries present with obvious deformity, especially the so-called Colles' fracture with its characteristic 'dinner fork' appearance, whereas others such as scaphoid fractures may have little obvious swelling, bruising or deformity. It is helpful to look at the wrist tangentially (i.e. sideways on) as subtle abnormalities may only be detected this way. Always compare with the other limb. Visually identify anatomical landmarks such as radial and ulnar styloid processes and inspect the forearm bones up to and including the elbow. Use the wrist creases to identify the carpal bones. The scaphoid tubercle is usually easily identified as the bony prominence on the palmer aspect of the wrist (see Figure 6.1).

Feel

Ask the patient to point to the area of maximum tenderness, and then start the palpation away from this point working your way systematically towards it, ensuring the whole limb is examined. Pay particular attention to the scaphoid bone and the anatomical snuff box. The anatomical snuff box is found on the lateral aspect of the wrist when the thumb is extended, and is formed by the tendons of abductor pollicis longus, extensor pollicis brevis and extensor pollicis longus (see Figure 6.2). On the floor of the box lie the radial styloid, scaphoid, trapezium and the base of the first metacarpal. Finally, ensure a full neurovascular assessment is carried out.

Move

The forearm bones can rotate along their long axis in movements known as *supination* and *pronation* to enable re-alignments of the hand/finger. During supination, the forearm bones lie flat in their anatomical position, but during pronation the radius rotates its head while its distal end swings around the ulna, thus changing the hand position from palmer to dorsal. Fractures to the long bones can severely restrict supination/pronation.

The wrist movements can be confusing depending on whether the forearm is supinated or pronated. Remember the anatomical position: elbow fully extended and palm facing forward. It is from this position movements take place. The movements and their approximate degrees are:

- flexion = 75°
- extension = 75° (this is commonly described as dorsi-flexion, although strictly speaking 'dorsi-flexion' is a movement of the foot)

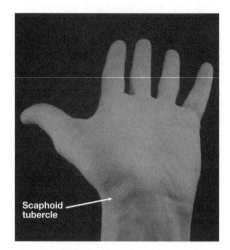

Figure 6.1 Scaphoid tubercle.

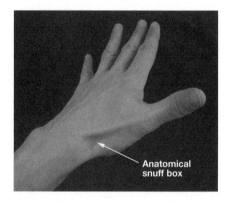

Figure 6.2 The position of the anatomical snuff box.

Abduction and adduction are hardly ever used to describe wrist movement. Instead, radial and ulnar deviation is used (20° and 35° respectively). Radial deviation is more resisted than ulna deviation due to the position of the radial styloid. The forearm and wrist have extensive muscle and tendon supply acting on the hand and fingers. It is outside the scope of this book to review them all, but as a *general* rule (there are a few exceptions) they can be divided into two groups (Dean and Pegington, 1996):

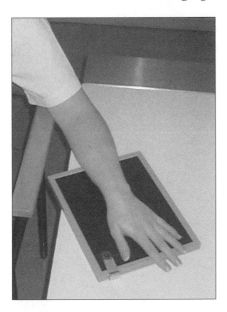

- **anterior (volar) surface:** the muscles and tendons lying at the front (anterior/volar aspect) of the forearm run into the palmer (volar) surface of the wrist and finger. Their main actions are pronation of the forearm and flexion of the wrist and fingers.
- **posterior (dorsal) surface:** the muscles and tendons lying at the back of the forearm run to the back of the wrist and hand. Their main actions are supination of the forearm and extension of the wrist and fingers.

Check all active and, depending on the patient's degree of pain and/or obvious deformity, also passive movements. Resisted movements should wait until you have ruled out any fractures and/or dislocation.

Standard projections

dorsi-palmer (DP) – this is, strictly speaking, a PA view
lateral

If a midshaft fracture is suspected, full radial and ulnar views should be requested. Bear in mind that these will project differently and demonstrate different anatomy and bony relationships, for this reason do not request radius and ulna when you mean wrist and vice versa.

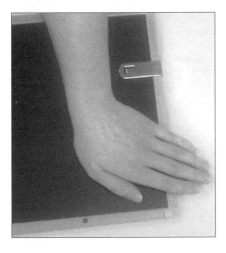

Figure 6.3 DP view of the wrist (top) and close-up of the DP scaphoid positioning (below) with ulnar deviation of the hand to better demonstrate the scaphoid.

Additional projections

oblique
scaphoid

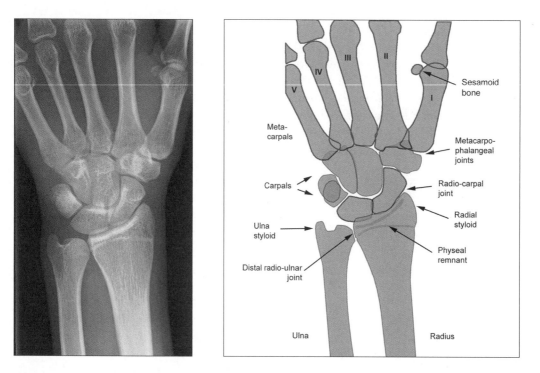

Figure 6.4 DP wrist view with a schematic diagram. The standard views should include the distal third of the radius and ulna and the metacarpals. The sclerotic line seen across the distal radius of this young adult patient is the remnant of the fusion of the radial shaft with the radial epiphyses, and this can often persist well into adulthood.

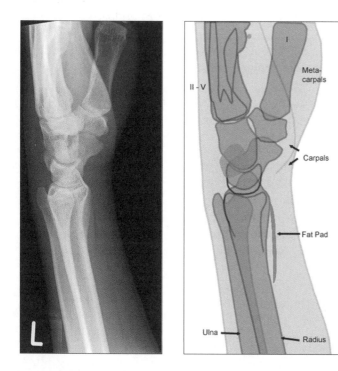

Figure 6.5 Lateral view with a schematic diagram. The curved black stripe on the lateral view volar to the distal radius is a useful soft-tissue sign if a fracture is not detected. This stripe is a layer of fat lying just anterior to the pronator quadratus muscle that is applied to the volar aspect of the distal radius and ulna. If it becomes effaced (obliterated) or bulges excessively, this is a sign of effusion within the wrist and the images should be carefully scrutinized again. It does not mean that there is definitely a fracture but that there has been significant trauma to the wrist. Note that this is not a perfectly positioned lateral view as the ulna is shown slightly dorsal to the radius, which means the wrist was slightly under-rotated when the image was taken. However, it is diagnostic and for the purposes of explanation it is easier to identify the anatomy of the individual bones when they are slightly separated.

X-ray positioning

To position for wrist views the patient sits sideways at the X-ray table and the beam is directed to a point midway between the radial and ulnar styloid processes. The wrist is then rotated onto its side, thumb uppermost, for the lateral view. If scaphoid views are required, imaging in ulnar deviation is preferred, i.e. the hand is turned away from the midline (ulnar deviation) in order to minimize any overlapping of the carpal bones. In the presence of a fracture, however, this can be extremely painful to achieve.

DP and lateral wrist views

The standard wrist views should include the distal third of the radial and ulnar shafts, the carpal bones and the metacarpals. Trace individually the cortex of all the long bones for fractures – common fracture sites are the distal radius, the ulnar styloid, the neck and base of the fifth metacarpal; although all the metacarpals are prone to fracture, the fifth does seem to be the more vulnerable. The distal articular surface of the radius should be scrutinized on the lateral view; it normally tips forward 10°–15° with respect to the long axis of the radius; variation from this indicates a fracture (but not necessarily a recent one).

It is important to know the carpal bones, their names, positions and approximate shape. Generally, the joint spaces around the carpals are uniform; so as well as examining each of these irregular bones for a fracture you must also examine the shape and the surrounding joint space. The ability to spot fractures and dislocations depends to a great

Figure 6.6
Radiograph with a schematic diagram of the carpal bones and associated articulations (sub-adult as the epiphyses are partially unfused). It is important to know the normal appearance of the carpals, as fractures, and in particular dislocations, are not always easy to spot. Note that in this individual there is negative ulnar variance, i.e. the ulna is slightly shorter than the radius, an example of a normal variant.

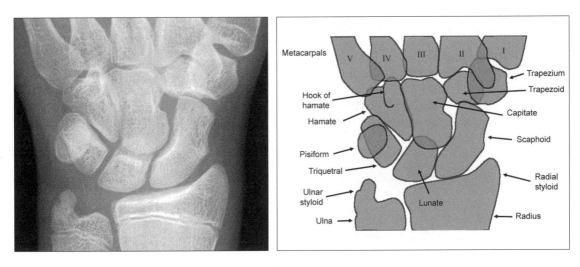

extent on knowing what is normal or what is a normal variation. This comes with time, experience, looking at lots of normal films and, unfortunately, probably making a few mistakes.

Normal alignments

When looking at wrist views, a useful tip is to check the angle of the articular surface of the distal radius with the radial shaft. It normally tips forward (towards the palm) by about 5°–10° from the horizontal (see Figure 6.7). Occasionally, the only apparent sign of a fracture is the absence or increase of this angle. Radial fractures that result in posterior angulation of the fragment are most common, and if you get into the habit of identifying the radial articular surface and checking it against the axis of the radial shaft you will find it assists in detecting subtle fractures. This angulation is also required, of course, in deciding whether a particular fracture requires manipulation or passive management only. Measuring the angulation is discussed in details under distal radial fractures.

Figure 6.7 Radiograph and schematic diagram of normal alignment from the lateral view. The angle of the radial articular surface should be checked against the long axis of the radial shaft. It normally tips forward by 5°–10° from the horizontal (see schematic). This can be a useful tool to identify fractures when no cortical break can be detected. It is important to be familiar with the normal alignment of the radius, lunate and capitate on the lateral view to identify subluxations or dislocations. Both these aspects of normal alignment are further discussed later in the chapter.

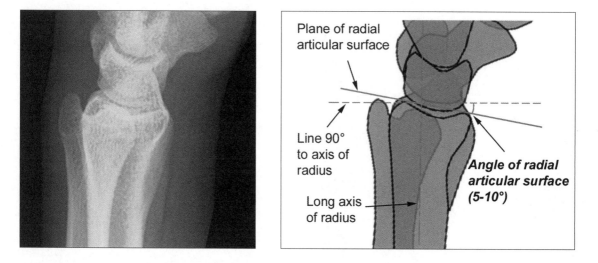

Plane of radial articular surface

Line 90° to axis of radius

Long axis of radius

Angle of radial articular surface (5-10°)

Common injuries

Injuries to the carpal bones

The mechanism of injury is usually a hyperextension or 'kick back' injury, commonly a fall onto the outstretched hand. Approximately 71% of all carpal bone fractures are to the scaphoid (McNally and Gillespie, 2004). Up to 50% of all scaphoid fractures occur to the waist, 38% to the proximal pole and 12% to the distal pole (McRae, 1999) – see Figure 6.8 – and there are far-reaching implications if the fracture is not adequately treated. The scaphoid receives its blood supply via arteries penetrating the distal pole only. In a fracture of the scaphoid waist, the distal pole will maintain its blood supply and therefore receive oxygen and nutrients for repair to take place. However, the blood supply to the proximal pole is likely to have been interrupted by the fracture, and there exists a potential for avascular necrosis, where healing of the fracture fails and the bone effectively dies. An example of this is shown in Figure 6.13.

There is not one single test that can positively exclude a fracture. If a scaphoid fracture is clinically suspected, the procedures followed to confirm the injury tend to vary between institutions. A scaphoid fracture, particularly if it is absolutely undisplaced, may not show on initial X-ray at the time of injury. If the wrist is subsequently X-rayed again ten days post-injury and there is a fracture present, a certain amount of bone healing will have taken place; this includes reabsorption of bone at the fracture site that therefore widens the fracture and renders it visible on the radiograph. In some institutions, wrist X-rays only are done at the time of injury and then (assuming no abnormality is seen) X-rayed again with a scaphoid series after ten days, by which time any fracture should be apparent. The initial treatment of a suspected scaphoid injury is therefore by clinical findings, and you

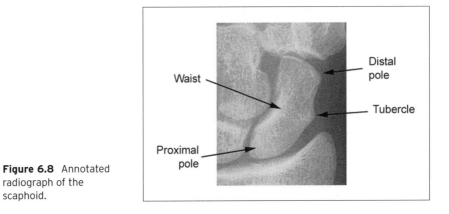

Figure 6.8 Annotated radiograph of the scaphoid.

would be negligent in not treating such an injury as fractured, regardless of the initial X-ray findings.

There is often no bruising, deformity and only minimal swelling in
scaphoid injuries, although localized swelling in the anatomical snuff
box might be present (McRae, 1999). If diffuse swelling, bruising and
deformity are seen, suspect another injury such as dislocation of the
carpal bones. There will be localized tenderness over the injured carpal
bone, and the scaphoid tubercle (see Figure 6.1) should be palpated on
the dorsal and palmer aspect simultaneously. The anatomical snuff
box must be pressed (see Figure 6.2) and compared with the other
wrist as the anatomical snuff box is normally tender (McNally and
Gillespie, 2004). These two tests are probably the most useful in deter-
mining scaphoid tenderness, but other fractures may also produce
pain. Check the neurovascular status distally. Wrist movements can be
severely restricted and/or painful depending on the degree of bony and
ligamentous injury. The scaphoid should be evaluated using the axial
(scaphoid) compression test (also known as telescoping the thumb into
the snuff box) – see Figure 6.9. The thumb is pushed down into the
anatomical snuff box compressing the scaphoid between the first
metacarpal (and trapezium) and the radius. If there is a fracture present, the patient will complain of pain in the wrist.

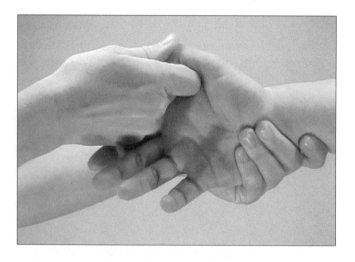

Figure 6.9 Telescoping the thumb using the axial compression test
for scaphoid fracture.

Scaphoid views

A scaphoid series normally comprises four views, although again this can vary with local protocols: dorsi-palmer (DP), DP cranial angulation, DP oblique and a lateral (see Figure 6.10). In order to reduce the superimposition of adjacent bones, the scaphoid views are taken with the wrist in ulnar deviation, i.e. the palm of the hand flat on the cassette is turned away from the patient. However, in the presence of a fracture the patient may strongly object to this.

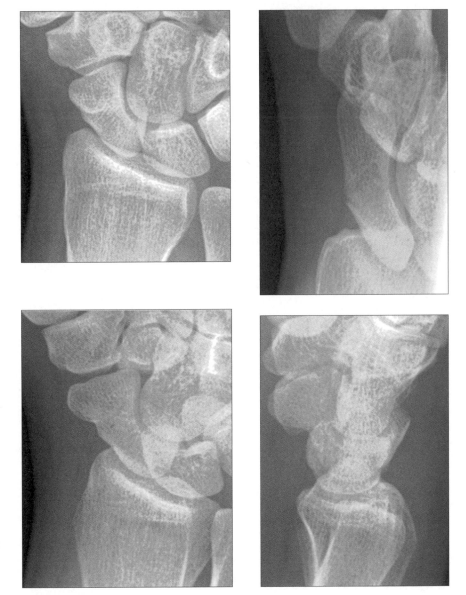

Figure 6.10 Scaphoid series – DP (top left), DP cranial angulation (top right), DP oblique (bottom left) and lateral (bottom right). The top two views demonstrate the scaphoid waist and associated articulations well, and the oblique view demonstrates the distal pole. Any one of these views can be the only one to show a fracture in a patient; therefore, careful scrutiny of each one is required.

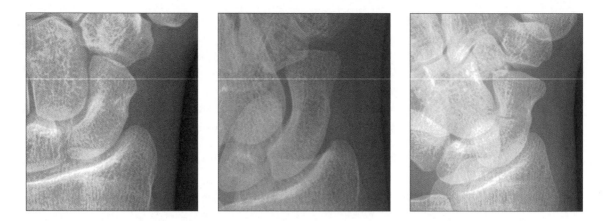

Figure 6.11 A classic fracture of the scaphoid waist. Note that it is only clearly shown on the oblique view. The scaphoid is a particularly irregularly shaped bone, which is why so many views are required. Scaphoid fractures are extremely rare in sub-teen children as all the carpals are surrounded by a thicker layer of cartilage than in the adult; this is protective as the cartilage is more flexible than bone.

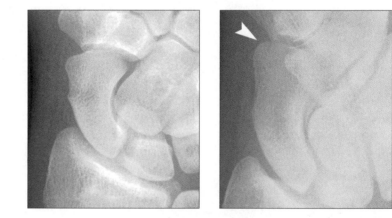

Figure 6.12 An unusual fracture of just the tip of the distal pole of the scaphoid, this time only visible on the DP angulated view (arrowhead).

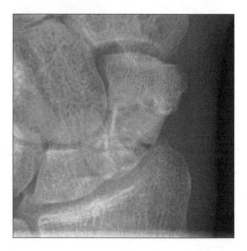

Figure 6.13 Avascular necrosis. The scaphoid fracture has failed to heal adequately and the proximal half of the scaphoid has undergone a breakdown of the normal bone tissue as that part of the bone has been denied adequate oxygen and nutrient supplies to allow effective bone healing. Note the coarsened trabecular pattern and the lack of normal cortex. In time, this is likely to give further problems as degenerative changes are accelerated.

Treatment

Fractures are treated with the standard scaphoid plaster – which is below-elbow, wrist-neutral and with a slight radial deviation (or neutral) – for approximately six weeks. Many orthopaedic textbooks recommend additional immobilization of the thumb up to the inter-phalangeal joint, but this is now disputed, as the function is unnecessarily restricted (McNally and Gillespie, 2004). The treatment of clinically but radiologically negative fractures is slightly more controversial. The usual practice of immobilizing the patient in the standard scaphoid plaster of Paris is disputed as fractures that do not show initially are stable and have a good prognosis (McNally and Gillespie, 2004). Many centres now use a splint (e.g. Futuro) or elasticated tubular bandage as support and pain relief until the patient is reviewed.

Other carpal fractures

The following images are all fractures of carpal bones other than the scaphoid. It must be pointed out that, with the possible exception of the triquetral, fractures of these bones are extremely rare. Nevertheless, all the bones of the wrist should be carefully and methodically examined on the radiograph to ensure a fracture is not missed.

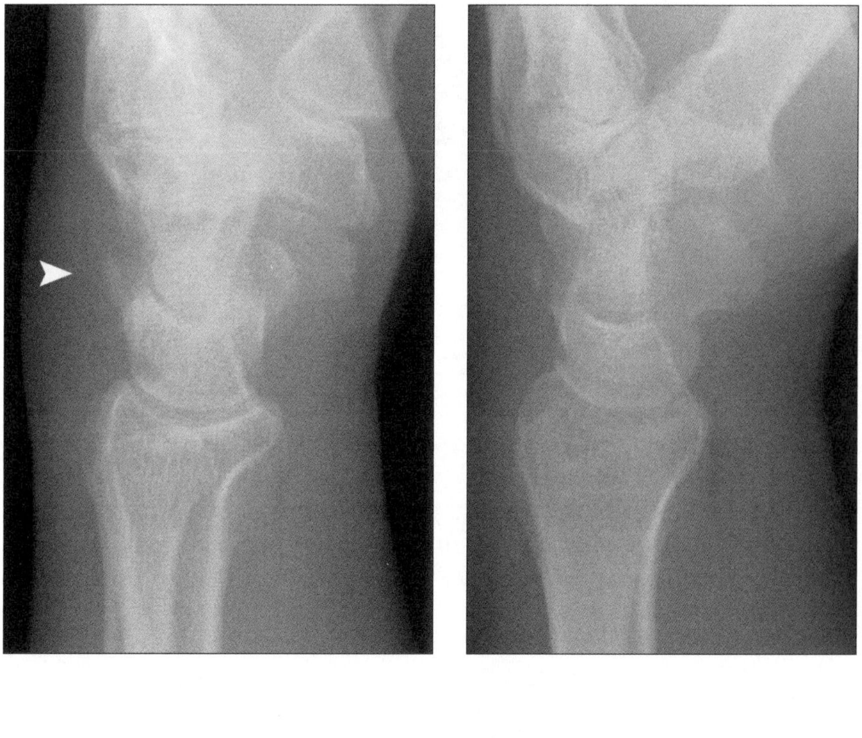

Figure 6.14 Two examples of triquetral 'flake' fractures. A flake of bone becomes avulsed from the dorsum of the triquetral and is seen as a separate fragment from the rest of the carpals. The DP view is almost always normal (not shown). This is probably the next-most-common carpal fracture after the scaphoid but is often missed on the initial examination of the films. Treatment is as for soft-tissue injury and should not be immobilized. A splint/bandage may be given for pain relief.

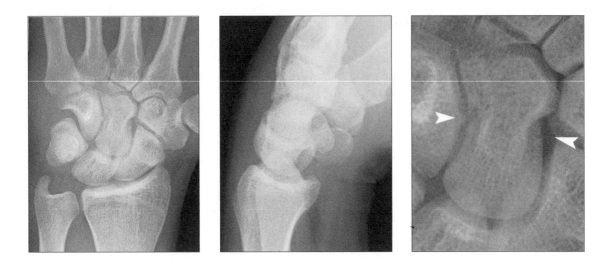

Figure 6.15 Fracture of the capitate. This is very easy to miss, but the fracture is visible. Always have a magnifying glass or use the magnifying tools on a viewer workstation to ensure these fractures are detected (arrowheads). Treatment is six weeks' immobilization in a plaster cast, less for avulsion fractures.

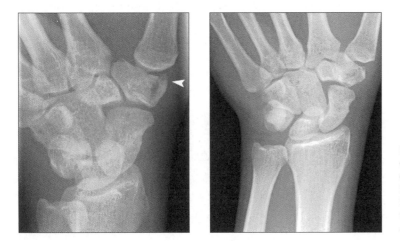

Figure 6.16 This is the only example of a trapezium fracture that we have come across; however, if it is a bone, it can fracture and so we decided to include it in the text. Treatment is six weeks' immobilization in a plaster cast, less for avulsion fractures.

Dislocations

Several ligaments hold all the carpal bones tightly together. On the DP view, the spaces between the carpal bones are equal and should not be more than 2 mm wide. Severe ligamentous injury can lead to the rupture of these ligaments and a subsequent dislocation of all carpal bones, but the most common are:

- scapho-lunate dislocation

- lunate dislocation
- peri-lunate dislocation

These injuries are rare but carry a high risk of neurovascular complications. They are often overlooked, which can be avoided by checking the normal alignment of the bones. Obvious deformity is rarely seen, but there is usually significant swelling.

Scapho-lunate dislocation

A widening gap (known as the 'Terry-Thomas' sign after the English actor who had a famously wide gap between his two front teeth) is seen between the scaphoid and lunate. An associated fracture of the scaphoid may also be present. Refer these injuries to orthopaedics for manipulation under image intensifier or for the surgical repair of the ligaments.

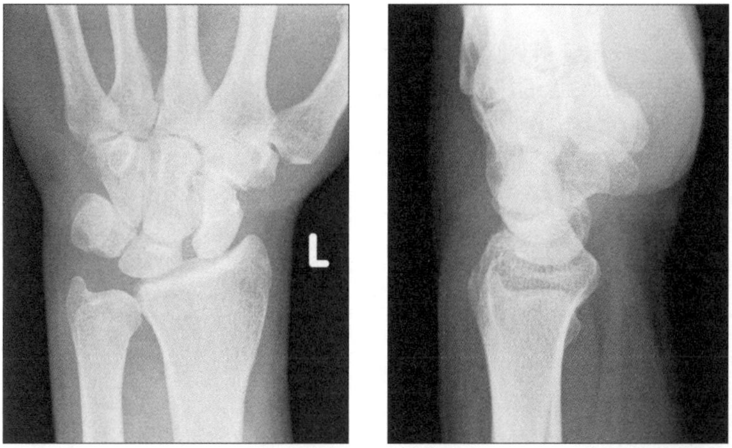

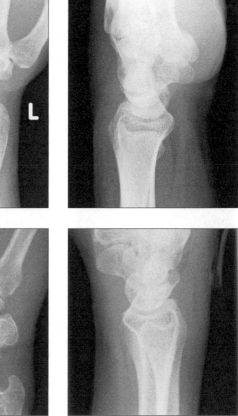

Figure 6.17 Careful scrutiny of these images reveals no fracture. However, look again at the joint spaces around the carpals: there is a wider gap than normal between the lunate and scaphoid indicating scapho-lunate ligament disruption.

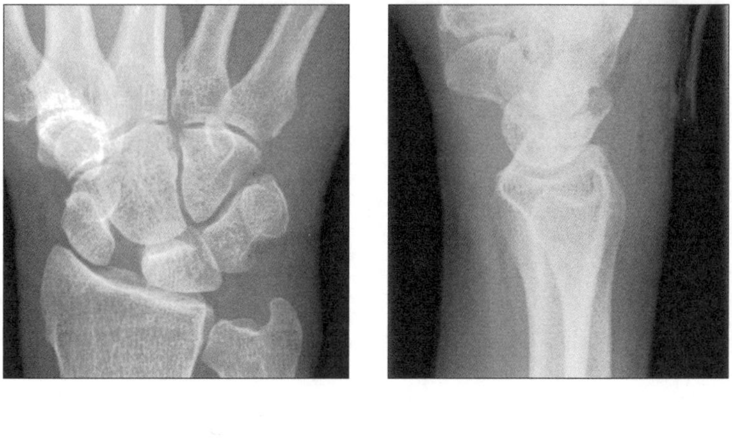

Figure 6.18 Another 'Terry-Thomas' sign with a clearly widened scapho-lunate joint space. In this example, the disruption is so severe that the scaphoid has rotated in the dorsi-plantar plane giving the distorted appearance seen in the DP view (left). The lateral view (right) is normal.

Lunate and peri-lunate dislocations

As previously stated, on the lateral view, the distal radius, lunate and the capitate lie in a straight line and articulate with each other.

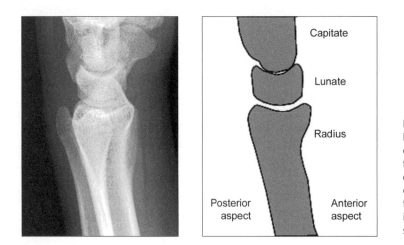

Figure 6.19 When examining the lateral view, check for subluxations or dislocations: the lunate sits within the dished articular surface of the distal radius and, in turn, the capitate sits within the concavity of the upper border of the lunate. This is illustrated in the simplified schematic diagram.

When the lunate dislocates, the capitate and the radius remain in a straight line, but the lunate has slipped volarly so that it lies in front of the other carpal bones – see Figure 6.20 left (below). In a peri-lunate dislocation, the radius and lunate remain in a straight line, but the capitate dislocates – see Figure 6.20 right (below).

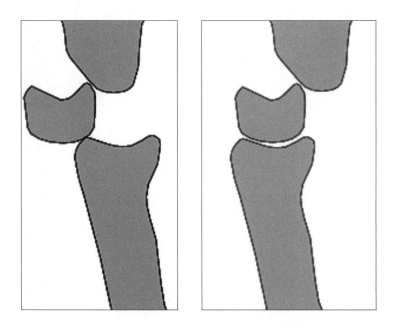

Figure 6.20 Lunate dislocation and peri-lunate dislocation. The lunate has dislocated posteriorly (left), but there is normal alignment between the radius and capitate. This time the lunate and radius remain in normal alignment (right), but the capitate has dislocated anteriorly.

Figure 6.21 This is a seriously injured wrist; on inspecting the DP view (left), the scaphoid fracture is immediately apparent. However, look carefully at the joint spaces around all the carpals; the lunate is a strange shape and, on looking at the lateral view (right), it becomes apparent that it is partially dislocated anteriorly together with the proximal pole of the scaphoid. Surgical intervention is required to reduce the dislocation and repair the scaphoid fracture.

Figure 6.22 In this second example of a wrist dislocation the appearance of the carpals is very abnormal on the DP view (left), and there is clearly a fracture of the scaphoid. On the lateral view (right), it becomes obvious that the capitate has dislocated from the lunate posteriorly and also migrated inferiorly along with the proximal pole of the scaphoid. Unlike the previous example in Figure 6.21, the lunate remains in articulation with the distal radius. This is a peri-lunate dislocation. Refer to orthopaedics for surgical intervention.

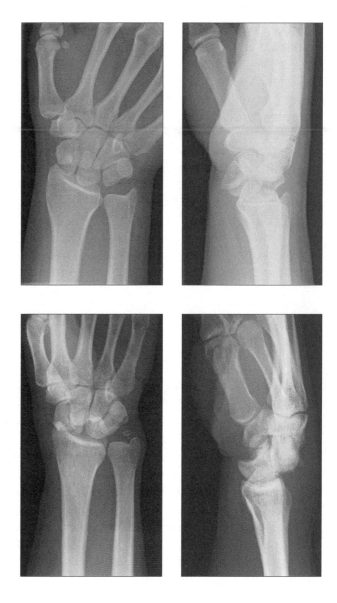

Fractures to the distal radius/ulna

Fractures to the distal radius usually occur as a result of a fall onto the outstretched or, more rarely, onto the dorsum of the hand with the wrist in flexion (Dandy and Edwards, 2003). Different patterns of injury occur, many of which have very familiar names taken from the surgeons who first described them. However, this familiarity is often of a disservice when interpreting a radiograph as the fractures can be mistaken or not fully understood. It is far more accurate and prevents a lot of confusion (and potential embarrassment if mistaken) just describing what is seen. We will utilize some of these names here but only as they are so familiar in clinical practice and will aid readability. We must point out that in our own clinical practice we would never report on an X-ray using names of surgeons – we would always describe what is found.

If the patient is in quite severe pain, they will guard the fracture by resting the injured wrist on the palm of the other hand. There is usually significant swelling and deformity. The so-called Colles' fracture has a characteristic deformity described as a 'dinner fork'. Bruising may be present. Palpate shoulder, humerus and elbow and the shafts of the radius and ulna. Assess the carpal bones before finally palpating the distal radius and ulna. Ensure a full neurovascular assessment is carried out. The movements are significantly reduced and often the patient will usually resist any attempts to move the wrist.

Colles' fracture

The Colles' fracture is defined as: 'a fracture of the radius within 2.5 cm of the wrist with a characteristic deformity if present' (McRae, 1999: 314). It is most commonly seen in the over fifties, especially post-menopausal women owing to diminished bone density of osteoporosis (McRae, 1999; Dandy and Edwards, 2003).

It is probably the most common fracture seen in the A&E/MIU environment, accounting for between 10% and 20% of all fractures. The fracture was first described in 1814 in a treatise published in the *Edinburgh Surgical and Medical Journal* by the surgeon Abraham Colles, professor of anatomy and surgery in Dublin, and his name has been given to this injury ever since. It is noteworthy that this accurate description of the injury was written over eighty years prior to the discovery of X-rays.

On the radiograph, look for the following abnormalities, which may not all be present but must be looked for in order to determine the treatment:

Impaction: DP view, see Figure 6.23
Lateral (radial) displacement and radial angulation: DP view, see
    Figure 6.24
Dorsal displacement/angulation: lateral view, see Figure 6.25

Impaction

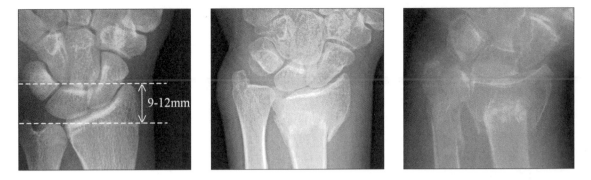

Figure 6.23 As a rule, the radial styloid sits 9–12 mm above the articular surface of the distal ulna (left). At the site of articulation with the lunate, the articular surfaces of the radius and ulna are on the same level (left). As the shaft of the radius impacts into the fragment, the length is reduced. Also note the increased density. The radius and ulna are no longer at the same level at the site of articulation of the lunate (centre and right). Often, the triangular cartilage is torn causing an associated avulsion fracture to the ulnar styloid (right).

Lateral (radial) displacement and radial angulation

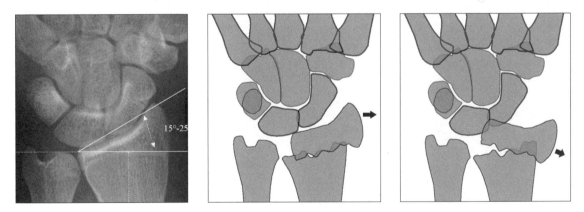

Figure 6.24 On the normal DP view (left), the radius has a 15°–25° tilt towards the ulna. The fragment slips into lateral (radial) displacement (centre) and may further tilt into radial angulation (right), losing the normal 15°–25° tilt towards the ulna. The tilt is measured by drawing a line at the level of the radio-ulnar articulation perpendicular to the axis of the radius. A second line connects the radial styloid process and the lower (ulnar aspect) end of the radius. The tilt can now be measured. Try and apply this principle to the right-hand image.

Dorsal displacement/angulation

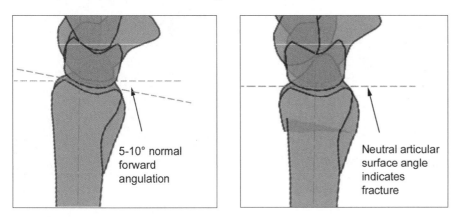

5-10° normal forward angulation

Neutral articular surface angle indicates fracture

Figure 6.25 Schematic diagram of a Colles' fracture. The diagram on the left shows the normal forward tilt of 5°–10° (see also Figure 6.7). In the Colles' fracture, if the force if sufficient, the fracture fragment tilts dorsally (backward) as demonstrated in the schematic diagram on the right. Dorsal displacement of more than 5° (i.e. a total of 10° from normal position) needs reduction.

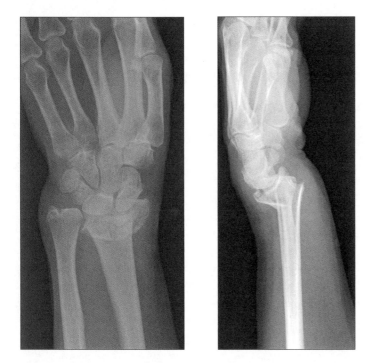

Figure 6.26 A Colles' fracture: amongst the most-common bone injuries seen in an A&E/MIU. The articular surface of the distal radius is tipped posteriorly, giving the characteristic 'dinner fork' deformity. The fracture is impacted, and there is also an undisplaced fracture of the ulnar styloid. In this case, treatment would include a reduction of the fracture to give adequate mobility. Try and draw the lines from Figures 6.23, 6.24 and 6.25.

Treatment

The treatment depends on degree of abnormalities. McRae (1999) suggests the following as indications for manipulation:

- obvious deformity on inspection
- marked radial angulation (other textbooks suggest < 10° loss of radial angle)
- > 5° of dorsal angulation
- impaction should be reduced as this will restrict normal movements.

Manipulation is usually undertaken under block (either haematoma or Biers') or sedation. General anaesthetic is generally reserved for younger people, failed reductions, old fractures (> 24 hours) and comminuted intra-articular fractures. The wrist is immobilized in a below-elbow back-slab. There are several methods described to reduce and correct Colles' deformities, but MacRae (1999) has a particular clear and helpful section of reduction method that the reader is advised to consult.

Smith's fracture

This is caused by a fall onto the dorsum of the hand with wrist in flexion and is sometimes referred to as a *reverse Colles'*.

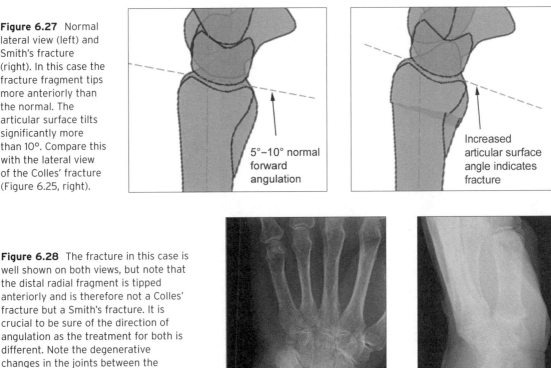

Figure 6.27 Normal lateral view (left) and Smith's fracture (right). In this case the fracture fragment tips more anteriorly than the normal. The articular surface tilts significantly more than 10°. Compare this with the lateral view of the Colles' fracture (Figure 6.25, right).

5°–10° normal forward angulation

Increased articular surface angle indicates fracture

Figure 6.28 The fracture in this case is well shown on both views, but note that the distal radial fragment is tipped anteriorly and is therefore not a Colles' fracture but a Smith's fracture. It is crucial to be sure of the direction of angulation as the treatment for both is different. Note the degenerative changes in the joints between the scaphoid and trapezium/trapezoid with loss of joint space and subsequent bony sclerosis.

Scrutinize the DP view for same pattern of abnormalities as a Colles' fracture. Differentiating between a Colles' and a Smith's fracture is only evident on the lateral view, where the fragment is displaced anteriorly (volar tilt).

Treatment

Smith's fractures are unstable. Manipulation is attempted usually under general anaesthetic but may need open reduction and internal fixation. They are immobilized in an above-elbow slab applied to the anterior surface of the arm, with the elbow flexed and the wrist extended.

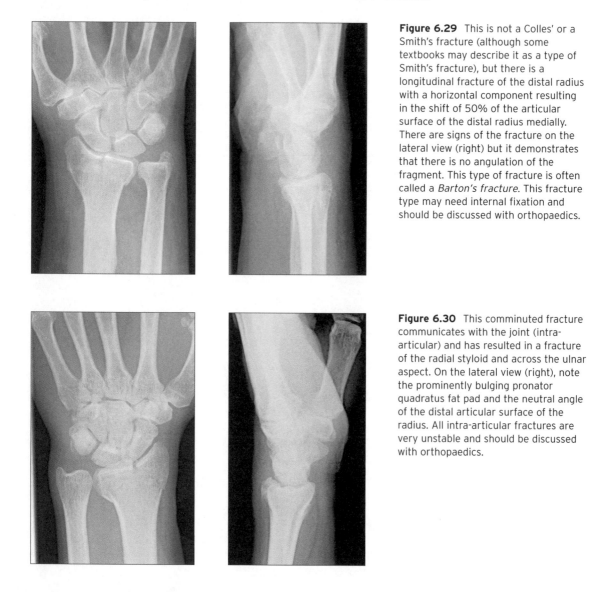

Figure 6.29 This is not a Colles' or a Smith's fracture (although some textbooks may describe it as a type of Smith's fracture), but there is a longitudinal fracture of the distal radius with a horizontal component resulting in the shift of 50% of the articular surface of the distal radius medially. There are signs of the fracture on the lateral view (right) but it demonstrates that there is no angulation of the fragment. This type of fracture is often called a *Barton's fracture*. This fracture type may need internal fixation and should be discussed with orthopaedics.

Figure 6.30 This comminuted fracture communicates with the joint (intra-articular) and has resulted in a fracture of the radial styloid and across the ulnar aspect. On the lateral view (right), note the prominently bulging pronator quadratus fat pad and the neutral angle of the distal articular surface of the radius. All intra-articular fractures are very unstable and should be discussed with orthopaedics.

Figure 6.31 Another longitudinal fracture of the distal radius intersecting the articular surface. This time the appearance is much more subtle. Damage to the articular surface is seen on the lateral view (right), although there is no angulation.

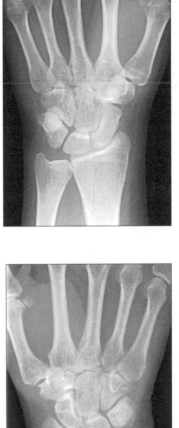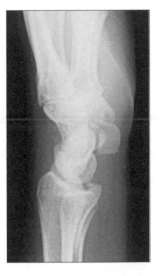

Figure 6.32 This is an extremely missable fracture of the distal radius. There is no discernible abnormal tilt of the distal articular surface (lateral view, top right). The fracture line on the DP is just visible – detail view (bottom left). The real clues are the prominently bulging fat pad and a break in the cortex posteriorly – black and white arrowheads respectively on the lateral detail view (bottom right). If there is doubt over the film and there is strong clinical suspicion of a fracture, a subsequent X-ray ten days post-injury will usually clarify one way or the other.

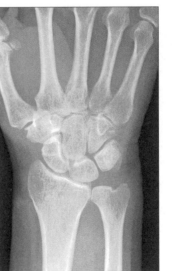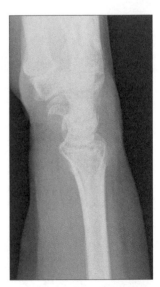

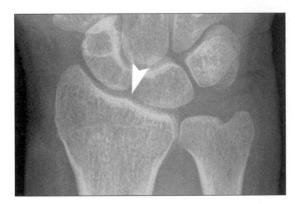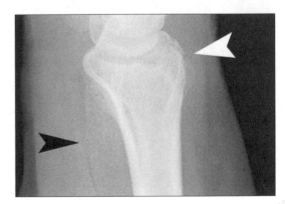

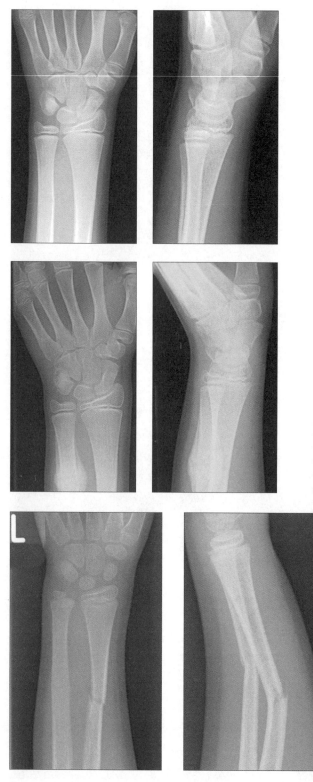

Figure 6.33 These images illustrate the point made in the previous case. The initial views of a boy's wrist following a fall are completely normal. The patient returned one month later and the resultant images are shown below (Figure 6.34). There is a transverse fracture of the ulnar shaft with exuberant callus formation due to the lack of immobilization at the time of injury. The normal remodelling process, over time, will re-absorb much of the excessive new bone growth.

Figure 6.34 Radial and ulnar views here demonstrate midshaft fractures in this juvenile patient. The AP view (left) belies the severity of the fracture angulation, which is only clearly shown on the lateral view (right). This demonstrates the importance of obtaining two views at 90º.

Figure 6.35 Another pair of angulated radial and ulnar shaft images. Again, the AP view (left) does not show the extent of the injury, which will require manipulation under anaesthesia. Note the classic 'dinner fork' deformity on the lateral view (right). Because of pain, the patient was unable to position conventionally for the examination. The radiographer has therefore annotated the lateral view to indicate non-standard positioning technique with a horizontal X-ray beam.

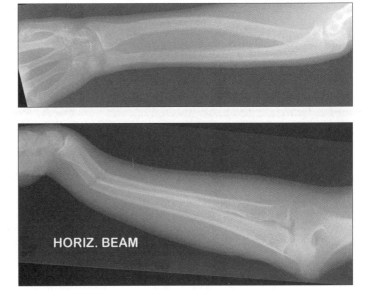

HORIZ. BEAM

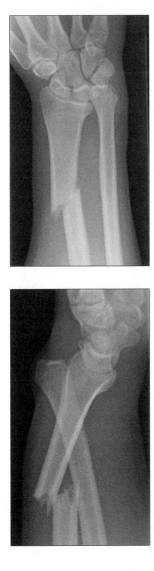

Fractures to the radial and ulnar shafts

Isolated fractures to the radial and ulnar shafts usually only occur as a result of direct violence (McRae, 1999). Likewise, it is rare for the distal radio-ulnar joint to be dislocated in isolation either – there is usually a fracture to the shaft of the radius.

The so-called Galeazzi's fracture dislocation (see Figure 6.36) is a fracture to the shaft of the radius with dislocation of the distal radio-ulnar joint. This injury should not be confused with a fracture to the shaft of the ulna and a dislocation of the radial head. This type of injury is know as a Monteggia's fracture/dislocation and is discussed in Chapter 5, although an example is provided in Figure 6.37 for comparison. The mechanism of injury for both fracture-dislocations is a fall onto the outstretched hand.

Never accept a fracture to the shaft of the radius or ulna until you have positively ruled out a dislocation to the distal radio-ulnar joint (galeazzi's) or radial head (monteggia's).

Figure 6.36 Fracture to the radial shaft. On the lateral view (bottom), note the dislocation of the ulna at the radio-ulnar joint. This is a Galeazzi's fracture/dislocation.

Treatment

The treatment is usually open reduction and internal fixation as there is a high risk of 'slipping' in the plaster after successful manipulation (Dandy and Edwards, 2003). An above-elbow plaster cast is necessary, which is also the treatment for minimal/undisplaced radial or ulnar shaft fractures.

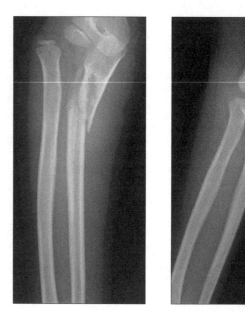

Figure 6.37 Fracture to the proximal ulna with a dislocation of the radial head. This is a Monteggia's fracture/dislocation.

Paediatric wrist injuries

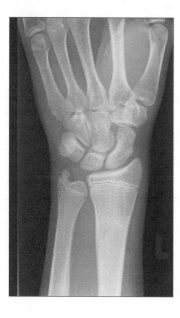

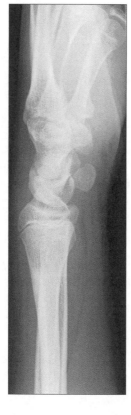

Figure 6.38 Looking at the lateral view (right), the radial articular surface is tipped posteriorly; however, no fracture line is detectable. On both views, a denser band is seen across the radial shaft, which is evidence of the healing of a previous fracture. Note that on the lateral view the pisiform is shown clear of the other carpal bones; this is a normal projectional artefact and demonstrates the position of the pisiform anterior to the triquetral.

Figure 6.39 This is a greenstick fracture in a young child with a clear fracture through one side of the cortex only. This is not classified as a Salter and Harris fracture as it does not involve the epiphysis. The child was in too much pain to position correctly for a true lateral view (left); however, the oblique view (right) thus obtained is diagnostic. Note that only four of the eight carpal bones are sufficiently mineralized to be radiopaque (which ones are missing?). A peculiarity of development of human metacarpals is that the first metacarpal has an epiphysis at the base or proximal end of the bone, whereas the second to fifth occur at the head or distal end. As this fracture is incomplete, with only one side of the cortex involved and no angulation, it will heal well in a below-elbow plaster cast and with orthopaedic follow-up.

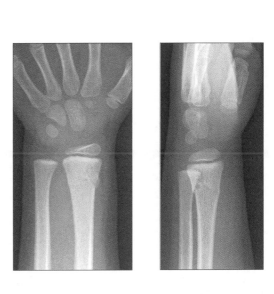

Figure 6.40 This example of a fracture in juvenile bone is called a torus fracture rather than a greenstick fracture as there is no break in the cortex. Instead, the cortex has buckled slightly; this type of fracture is often only detectable on the lateral view (right). Careful tracing of the cortex of the radius reveals the abnormal step just proximal to the epiphysis. As there is no angulation, treatment is conservative, with a below-elbow plaster cast for three to four weeks. (Note: *torus* means *protuberance* in Latin and is also an architectural term meaning a convex bulge at the base of a column, hence its use in describing this type of fracture.)

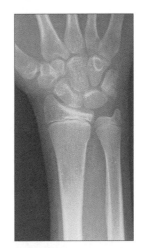
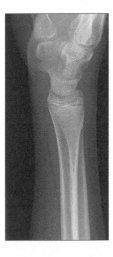

Figure 6.41 This is a slightly dorsally angulated bowing-type fracture of the distal radial and ulnar shafts. Also present at the fracture site is a thickening and blurring or greying of the cortex; this is bony callus formation and is indicative of a degree of healing having taken place. This image was obtained about two weeks post-injury when the child was still complaining of pain. This is a younger child than that of the previous example; only two carpals are clearly seen, while mineralization of the triquetral has just commenced.

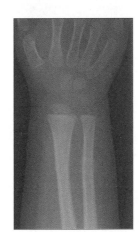
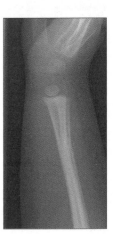

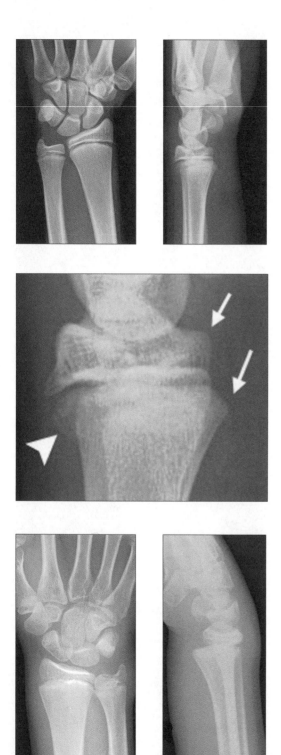

Figure 6.42a/b This is a more serious injury than the previous juvenile fractures seen as the fracture involves the epiphysis and will therefore affect the future bone growth if inappropriately treated. To work out the anatomy of the injury requires a careful scrutiny of the lateral view (right) and the tracing of the cortex of the individual bone shafts and epiphyses. In this case, the radial epiphysis has been displaced dorsally and retains a fragment of radial metaphysis, i.e. distal radial shaft. See also detail in Figure 6.42c below. Note that the radius on the DP view (left) appears completely normal but that there is an undisplaced fracture of the ulnar styloid.

Figure 6.42c Enlarged detail of the fracture of Figure 6.42b above (right). There is a misalignment of the margins of the radial epiphysis and metaphysis (arrows), and a fragment of metaphysis is still attached to the epiphysis (arrowhead), defining this as a Salter and Harris type II fracture. These fractures should be discussed with orthopaedic surgeons as they may need manipulation.

Figure 6.43 This fracture shows the displacement of the epiphysis posteriorly. No bone fragments are seen so this fracture is classified as a Salter and Harris type I fracture. The fracture is well shown on the lateral view (right), but note that on the DP view (left) the normally lucent physeal line separating the epiphysis from the metaphysis has been obliterated. This fracture can usually be treated in a below-elbow plaster cast and follow-up, but discuss with orthopaedics if unsure.

Carpal fractures in juveniles are very rare, particularly in sub-teenage children. The appearance in Figure 6.44 occasionally causes confusion. The pisiform is the last carpal bone to ossify and can often do so apparently in an irregular fashion. The pisiform on the lateral view is shown clear of the other carpals by a slightly over-rotated lateral projection, and it could easily be mistaken for an avulsed fragment of bone.

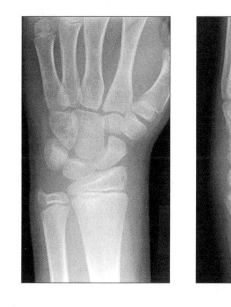

Figure 6.44 The irregularly ossifying pisiform in the lateral view (right) may be confused with an avulsion fracture. The key is to know where the pisiform is normally located and relate this to the known clinical history. Note that, unlike the ossification of the elbow, the ossification of the carpal bones is not as conveniently predictable. However, the capitate is *always* first to ossify (at around 4 months) and the pisiform is *always* the last (at 11 years). This is where the rules end and ossification of the rest of the carpals is not in strict order.

Chapter 7
The hand and fingers

Review of core anatomy

The hand and fingers (phalanges) have a complex anatomy to enable us to engage in a huge variety of very specialized and diverse functions and so any incorrect treatment of a relatively minor injury can have severe consequences for the patient.

The hand consists of five long bones (the metacarpals), which are described as having a head (the 'knuckles), shaft and a base (see Figure 7.5). The metacarpals articulate at their heads with the fingers at the metacarpo-phalangeal joints, and at the base with the carpal bones at the carpo-metacarpal joint (Figure 7.5). The metacarpals can be either named (e.g. 'ring finger' metacarpal) or numbered, with the thumb metacarpal being the first.

The fingers are always named (thumb, index, middle, ring and little fingers) and never numbered. Each finger consists of three bones: the distal, middle and proximal phalanges, with a proximal (PIP) and a distal inter-phalangeal joint. The thumb consists of a distal and a proximal phalanx only and one inter-phalangeal joint. To prevent confusion in identifying the correct side of the finger regardless of anatomical position, lateral and medial border is not used; instead, the terms radial ('thumb side') and ulna ('little-finger side') is applied.

The anatomical position of the hand is with the palm facing forward, and is referred to as either the palmer, volar or anterior aspect. The back of the hand is the posterior but is also referred to as dorsal aspect.

Clinical examination

As the hand is so important to everyday living, the patient's hand dominance, occupation and hobbies must be recorded as this can influence the treatment and prognosis (Guly, 1996). The principle of treatment is to restore as near optimum function as possible, which may still leave the patient with some degree of deformity. A thorough history is important, and, if the patient is able to do so, it is useful to place the injured hand in the position it was in when injured to anticipate possible damage (Wilson et al., 1997).

Look

The inspection must always be undertaken comparing the injured hand with the opposite hand. Note any bruising or swelling – is it localized to one area or more diffuse? Are there any wounds? If so, assess depth and thoroughly evaluate tendons and nerves. Observe for any obvious deformity – phalanges commonly dislocate. Look at the fingers 'end on' with the metacarpo-phalangeal joints flexed at 90°. The nails should be orientated in the same direction. When the fingers are fully flexed (at the proximal inter-phalangeal joints), they should all point towards the scaphoid, but always compare with the opposite hand. Fractures can cause mal-rotation ('scissoring') of a finger and the normal alignment/direction is disturbed (see Figure 7.1). This is more noticeable during full flexion. Obvious rotational deformity should be discussed with orthopaedic surgeons.

Figure 7.1
Observations of the fingers – 'end on' (left) and flexion of fingers (right), making the deformity more noticeable (Wardrope and English, 1998). (Reproduced by kind permission of Oxford University Press)

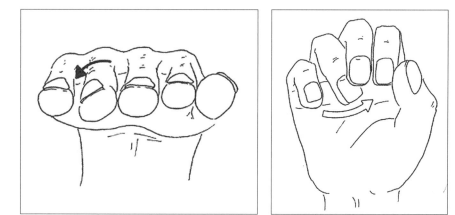

Feel

The aim is to identify the point of maximum tenderness and any other injuries that the patient may not have noticed to enable the correct radiograph to be obtained. Assessment of neurovascular status must be undertaken for even the most minor injury.

The hand receives its sensory supply from three nerves (two of which also provide motor branches): median, ulnar and radial. Sensation is tested by touching the finger and asking the patient if it feels the same throughout the digits and in comparison with the opposite hand. Do not simply ask the patient: 'Can you feel this?', as the patient is likely to say yes and not comment on any deficits (Guly, 1996). Alternatively, the digits are observed for sweating by rolling a pen gently down the side of the digit. Some resistance should be felt. If a nerve is completed severed, sweating will stop after about four minutes and no resistance will be felt (Wilson et al., 1997). This may be a useful test to use in the young child. Both these tests are useful for a rapid, generalized assessment, but a more specific test must be undertaken if any discrepancies are noted, and the two-point discrimination is recommended. A paper-clip is bent so that the ends can be opened or closed a varying distance from each other. Normal discrimination is a distance between the two ends of 6 mm apart when the two ends are applied to the finger, but some patients can tell the difference down to 3 mm. Discrimination only occurring over 6 mm is significant of injury.

The hand and fingers receive their vascular supply from the radial and ulnar arteries (both terminal branches of the brachial artery) on the palmer aspect. The arteries subdivide into several branches, some of which anatomize to form an arch. This collateral circulation ensures that when one artery has been divided (e.g. from trauma), the circulation is not impaired (Dandy and Edwards, 2003). Each finger receives a palmer digital artery to each side of the finger running alongside the digital nerve.

Move

There are several specialist movements taking place in the hand and fingers, some of which are outside the scope of this book. The metacarpo-phalangeal joints flex approximately 90° and has a hyper-extension of 30°. The inter-phalangeal joints are all capable of flexion and extension. The fingers (except the middle finger) all adduct and abduct towards and away from the middle finger. The thumb, in addition to the above, also has opposition with the little finger and circumduction.

Start with assessing the overall function of the hand and fingers, by asking the patient to make a fist and then straighten the hand and fingers, noticing areas of deficits that should then be assessed in more depth. The hand and fingers have an extensive and complex supply of tendons and it is outside the scope of this book to discuss them all. However, three structures are essential to be familiar with when interpreting radiographs: volar plate, extensor tendon and collateral ligaments.

On the palmer aspect of the fingers, the joints are stabilized by a thickening of the joint capsule known as the volar plate limiting hyper-extension (see Figure 7.2). The stability of the volar plate is tested by stabilizing the proximal phalanx and passively hyperextending the proximal inter-phalangeal joint. It should go no further or be more painful when compared to an uninjured joint.

Each finger has an extensor tendon terminating at the base of the distal phalanx. Over the proximal inter-phalangeal joint, the tendon has a broad expansion covering the dorsum of the proximal inter-pha-langeal joint. A unique feature of this expansion is that two additional muscles (lumbricals and interossei) insert into here. The extensor tendon can rupture off its distal phalanx insertion point resulting in a characteristic 'Mallet' finger deformity, where the patient is unable to extend the distal inter-phalangeal joint. As associated avulsion fracture may be present, but not always so, it is important to recognize this abnormality regardless of radiological findings.

The fingers and the thumb have two collateral ligaments covering the inter-phalangeal and metacarpo-phalangeal joints on the radial and ulnar border and are named accordingly. They stabilize the joint and restrict movements.

Figure 7.2 Stabilizing structures of the finger (Wardrope and English, 1998). (Reproduced by kind permission of Oxford University Press)

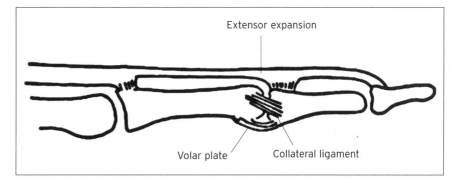

Avulsion fractures caused by a complete rupture of any of these structures are identified on the radiograph at the following points/view:

Table 7.1 Radiological appearance of fracture sites of stabilizing structures of the finger

Structure	Insertion point	X-ray view	Bony fragment site
volar plate	palmer aspect lying over inter-phalangeal joints	lateral	palmer aspect (see Figure 7.13)
extensor tendon	base of the distal phalanx	lateral	dorsal aspect (see Figure 7.14)
collateral ligaments	covers joints on the radial and ulna border	dorsi-palmer or lateral	lateral or medial (see Figure 7.11 and 7.12)

Standard projections

for fingers – dorsi-palmer (DP) and true lateral
for hand – DP and DP oblique

Additional views

A lateral hand is useful for foreign-body localization or to quantify fracture angulation but is not useful in fracture detection as there is a considerable overlap of bony structures

X-ray positioning

This is straightforward with the patient sitting sideways at the X-ray table and the hand placed on the cassette as shown for the DP oblique view positioned in Figure 7.3. The hand is positioned and immobilized using foam pads and sandbags as necessary. If a specific finger is of interest, this should be requested rather than hand views, as subtle finger fractures are not always well shown on the oblique hand projection. Even when the patient is in severe pain, diagnostic positioning is almost always achievable with a co-operative patient.

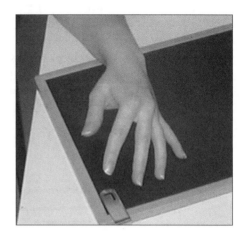

Figure 7.3 DP oblique view of the hand.

Radiographic interpretation

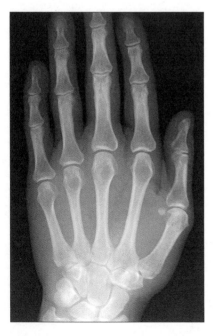

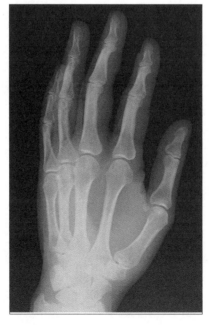

Figure 7.4 Normal hand views DP (left) and DP oblique (right). The thumb should be seen in true lateral on the DP view and shown in true AP on the oblique view. In practice, however, this is rarely the case and some degree of obliquity is usually seen. This is not a good projection to demonstrate subtle fractures of the fingers, which should be requested individually.

Figure 7.5 Schematic diagram of the DP radiograph in Figure 7.4.

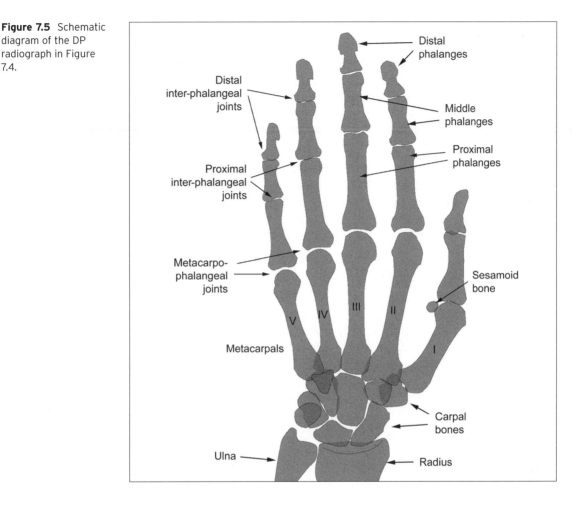

When looking at a radiograph of the hand, always bear in mind that these are compromise views: it is not possible to get two useful projections at 90°, owing to the amount of overlap and superimposition of the anatomy, but they do demonstrate the metacarpals well. These are complicated views; there are 29 individual named bones in the hand including the carpals and the distal radius and ulna; so a methodical approach to searching for fractures is required. Trace all the way around the cortex of each metacarpal; the articulations with the carpals are complex and the shape of the base of each metacarpal is irregular, but eliminate any wide joint spaces that might indicate a metacarpal dislocation. Note that there are usually several sesamoid bones around the metacarpo-phalangeal joints that should not be confused with avulsion fractures; they are smooth and rounded and lie within a tendon to resist wear. Pay particular attention to each metacarpal head, subtle punch-type injuries are occasionally missable here.

Check the congruity of the metacarpo-phalangeal joints; although dislocations of these joints are uncommon. Trace around the cortex of each phalanx, remembering that fractures of a finger are better shown with a true lateral (see Figure 7.9). In children metaphyseal fractures at the base of the proximal or middle phalanges are common and can be very subtle. Occasionally, a nutrient foramen may be seen on a radiograph of the phalanges, and if they are prominent they can be mistaken for a fracture (see Figure 7.6). A nutrient artery passes through the cortex via the foramen into the trabecular bone, and this is seen as a line crossing the cortex. It is distinguished from a fracture because it is greyer than a fracture line and it fans out slightly as it reaches the inner cortical boundary. Additionally, it only crosses one cortex, whereas a fracture will usually break the opposite side as well.

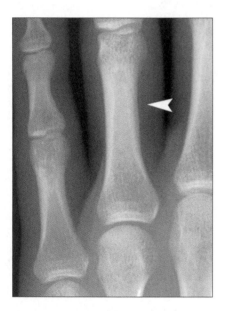

Figure 7.6 Nutrient foramen. A nutrient artery passes through the cortex of a long bone via a nutrient foramen in order to provide an arterial supply to the bone tissue. The foramen is seen as an oblique line crossing the cortex that usually fans out slightly as it crosses the inner border of the cortex (arrowhead). It is greyer than a fracture line as it does not cross the entire depth of the bone in the same way that a fracture does, and it also only crosses one cortex.

Radiographs of children's hands are more complex as there is an epiphysis for each metacarpal and for each phalanx (see Figure 7.9), which effectively doubles the number of bones to look at. The metacarpals of the fingers have an epiphysis at the distal end whereas the thumb has an epiphysis at the proximal end; however, an accessory epiphysis at the distal end also is not uncommon (see Figure 7.10). The carpal bones ossify in a regular sequence beginning with the capitate and ending with the pisiform. As mineralization progresses, the carpals take on the adult form but in intermediate stages can look irregular and be mistaken for fractures. Fractures of the fingers are less common than in adults but an injury involving a growth plate can lead to long-term complications if not treated correctly.

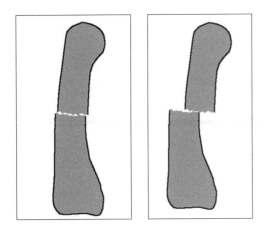

Figure 7.7 Fracture displacement as seen on DP view (left) shows almost no displacement; medial displacement (right) is 50%.

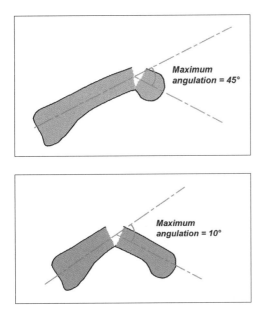

Maximum angulation = 45°

Maximum angulation = 10°

Figure 7.8 Site and angle of fracture angulation. The degree of acceptable angulation will depend on the site of the fracture. In the top image, the fracture is to the head of the metacarpal. In these injuries, an angulation of 45° or above needs referral. In the bottom image, the fracture is to the shaft, and here only an angulation of 10° or less is acceptable. You should consult your local guidelines or a standard orthopaedic textbook, such as McRae (1999), for specific guidance.

Finally, scrutinize the radiograph for normal alignment to detect and then measure deformities caused by a fracture. While measurement of displacement and angulation is important in all fractures, it is more so in the hand and fingers. The principles of measuring these deformities is discussed in the introduction to Part II (above) but is repeated here as it is such a significant feature in the management of hand and finger injuries.

Displacement

When a fracture is displaced, the bone ends have shifted in relation to each other and are described according to the movement of the distal fragment. Orthopaedic surgeons may at times measure the percentage of displacement, but in A&E/MIU, minimal, moderate or severe displacement is usually sufficient. Severe displacement must be corrected by manipulation (reduction), otherwise a shortening of the limb occurs.

Angulation

Of even greater importance in fracture management is the degree of angulation. To measure angulation, draw one line through the midline of the shaft. A second line is then drawn through the midline of the fragment – the angle can now be measured (see Figure 7.8).

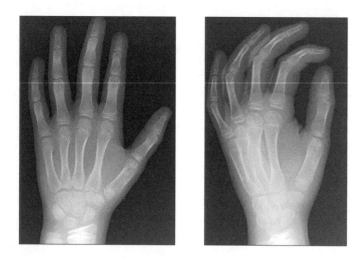

Figure 7.9 Paediatric hand views (10-year-old). Note the reversed first metacarpal with the epiphysis at the base. In this patient, there is also an accessory epiphysis at the head of the first metacarpal. This phenomenon is more clearly shown in Figure 7.10 of another patient. This appearance should not be confused with a fracture, as the margins are clearly smooth and rounded.

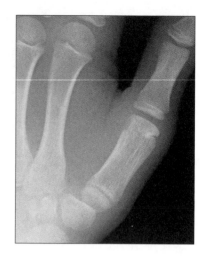

Figure 7.10 Fusing or partial accessory epiphysis at the distal first metacarpal. The primary epiphysis at the base is much more distinct and unfused.

Fractures/dislocations of the fingers and thumb

Fingers are easily injured and commonly dislocate. Mechanisms of injury include hyperextension (with or without twisting movements), crushing or forced flexion (e.g. stubbing finger). Following fractures or dislocations, joint stiffness occurs, which can be quite disabling and intensive physiotherapy may be required. Dislocations are usually obvious, although severe swelling may mask other injuries. It is usually due to a hyperextension injury and thus dislocates posteriorly. Post dislocation, swelling may continue for up to two years or never completely subside (Dandy and Edwards, 2003). Observe for any rotational deformity (see Figure 7.1). Avulsion fractures occur as a result of a rupture of the collateral ligament, volar plate or extensor tendon. Identify the point of maximum tenderness and state this on the X-ray request form to enable the radiographer to obtain optimal projection. Assess neurovascular status distally and ensure this is undertaken both before and after any reduction. The range of movements is severely restricted, but active flexion and extension should be assessed as this will help pinpoint areas of injury. Passive movements are best left until X-ray has ruled out any fractures.

Figure 7.11 Avulsion fracture. This is a typical undisplaced avulsion fracture at the base of the middle phalanx of the index finger caused by hyperextension. Excessive tension on the insertion of the collateral ligament has caused a small fragment of bone to separate and is visible as a fracture (arrowhead on detail view) on the lateral view. The DP view (left) is completely normal.

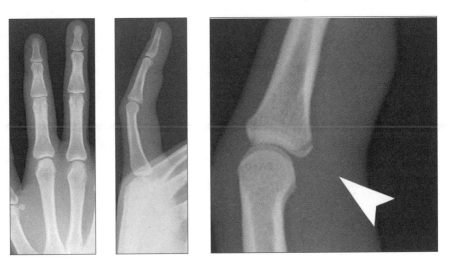

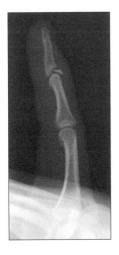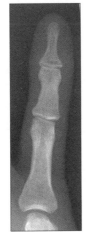

Figure 7.12 This is a more serious avulsion fracture with a greater degree of displacement and involvement of the articular surface. Again, the fracture is not clearly seen on the DP view (left).

Figure 7.13 An unusual and startling injury. This is a volar plate fracture where almost the entire cortex of the flexor aspect of the distal phalanx has been avulsed and migrated inferiorly. Note the absence of bony cortex as indicated by the arrowheads on the enlarged lateral view (right). The DP (left) view shows an area of increased density, which represents the fragment but is easily missed as it is superimposed over the middle phalanx. The fragment as seen on the lateral view (centre) could be mistaken for a penetrating foreign body.

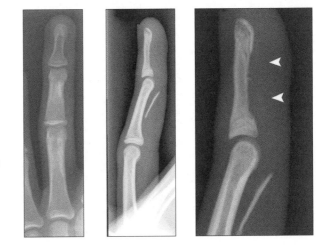

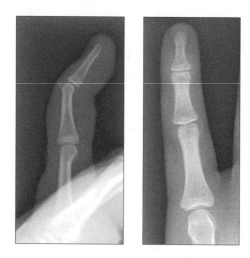

Figure 7.14 Mallet finger. A stubbing injury during a netball game has caused an avulsion fracture from the dorsal aspect at the base of the distal phalanx of this little finger. The extensor tendon has pulled the fragment of bone from the phalanx, and this has resulted in the characteristic forward droop of the tip of the finger.

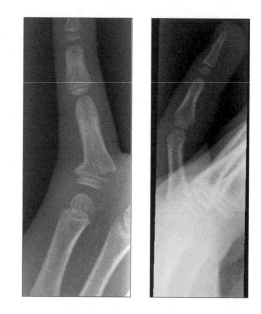

Figure 7.15 A markedly angulated metaphyseal fracture at the base of the proximal phalanx of the little finger. The fracture does not communicate with the growth plate itself.

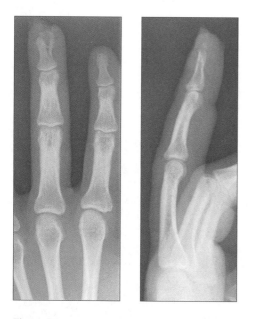

Figure 7.16 A vertical crush-type fracture that is both compound and comminuted. In this case, the seriousness of the injury is better shown on the DP view (left).

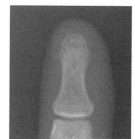

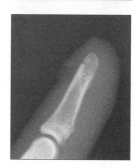

Figure 7.17 The patient was X-rayed in this case prior to relieving a subungual haematoma. There is a minimally displaced crush-type fracture of the distal phalanx. The elevation of the nail bed and soft-tissue damage can be seen, confirming that this is a compound fracture.

Figure 7.18 This is a comminuted fracture of the proximal phalanx resulting from a fall directly onto the thumb. The fracture angulation is shown on the lateral view (right), but there is no communication with the metacarpo-phalangeal joint.

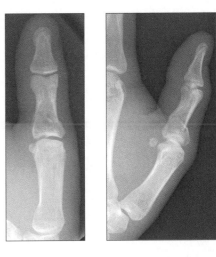

Figure 7.19 The DP view (left) of the ring and little fingers of this elderly gentleman following a fall shows some overlap of both proximal inter-phalangeal joints. The lateral views (centre) and (right) require careful scrutiny to work out the anatomy but reveal that the ring finger has a comminuted fracture at the base of the middle phalanx, while there is a dislocated proximal inter-phalangeal joint of the little finger.

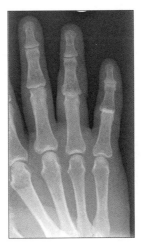
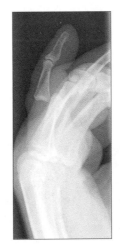
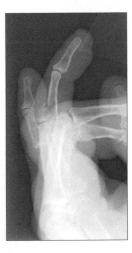

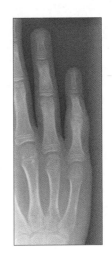
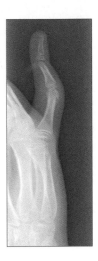

Figure 7.20 This fracture was also sustained following a fall. Note that the fracture communicates with the inter-phalangeal joint.

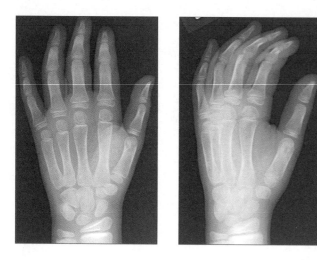

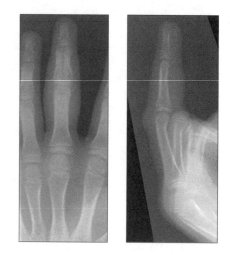

Figure 7.21 There are three metaphyseal fractures at the base of the proximal phalanges of the index, ring and middle fingers. The middle-finger injury is the most obvious, but do not assume that there is only one fracture; always scan the rest of the anatomy shown.

Figure 7.22 This is a Salter and Harris type II fracture of the middle phalanx of the middle finger (see Chapter 3 for an explanation of the Salter and Harris classification of fractures). This unusual vertical fracture extends from the distal articular surface to the growth plate at the base of the phalanx.

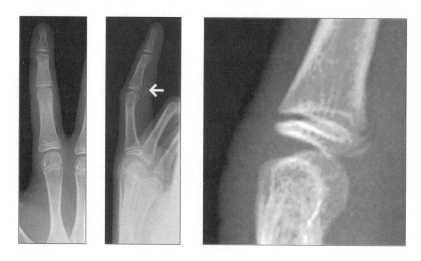

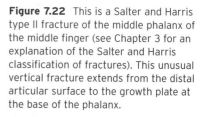

Figure 7.23 This image shows a subtle avulsion fracture at the base of the middle phalanx that affects both the epiphysis and the metaphysis and is therefore classified as a Salter and Harris type III fracture.

Treatment

The basic principle of treatment is to restore function as soon as possible to prevent joint stiffness. Fractures to the proximal phalanx are treated conservatively with pain relief and gentle exercise, although at times a splint may be used.

Undisplaced fractures to the proximal and middle phalanges are treated in neighbour strapping for two to four weeks, followed by physiotherapy. Angulation of > 10° should be reduced and then supported in flexion (McRae, 1999).

Dislocations are reduced by gentle traction. If muscle spasm is severe, insert a digital nerve block or use Entonox. Any failure to reduce once muscle spasm has been overcome is usually due to 'button-holing' of the phalanx head through the joint capsule, and open reduction is necessary. *Always* X-ray again post-reduction to check for alignment and any associated fractures. If no associated fractures are present, the finger is neighbour strapped for two weeks followed by physiotherapy.

Mallet finger deformity (with or without an associated avulsion fracture) must be placed in a special Mallet splint keeping the proximal inter-phalangeal joint straight but allowing movement of the distal inter-phalangeal joint. The patient should be advised that these injuries take a very long time to heal and the removal of the splint for cleaning must only take place with the finger supported in full extension.

All other avulsion fractures are usually treated by neighbour strapping, elevation and follow-up by orthopaedic/hand surgeons.

Metacarpal and thumb injuries

The most common metacarpal fracture is to the fifth metacarpal (may be known as a boxer's fracture) and is usually sustained by a punching injury with the metacarpal heads flexed in a fist, fracturing the neck. The shaft of fifth metacarpal fractures as a result of the little finger being twisted, whereas fractures to the second, third and fourth metacarpals usually occurs as a result of a twisting or crush injury (Dandy and Edwards, 2003).

The most common injury involving the thumb is a fracture through the base of the first metacarpal with or without a dislocation of the carpo-metacarpal joint, the presence of which is known as a 'Bennets fracture/dislocation'. The mechanism of injury is usually forced abduction or longitudinal force applied to the axis of the thumb (McRae, 1999), e.g. a boxing injury. The ulnar collateral ligament of the first metacarpal may rupture in forced abduction injuries. This injury is also known as *gamekeeper's thumb*. These days, it is a common injury sustained by skiers.

There is often extensive swelling especially if the hand is held dependently. Bruising may not be present initially. The hand is often held in partial flexion of the metacarpal heads. Observe for rotational deformity by noticing any scissoring of the fingers viewed 'end on'.

Note any wounds. These may be secondary to the hand punching a tooth thus converting the fracture into an open fracture with a high risk of infection. Tooth fragments have been known to be embedded in the hand. Identify the point of maximum tenderness but ensure the joint above and below is examined. There will be localized tenderness on the radial aspect of the first metacarpo-phalangeal joint in patients with ulnar collateral ligament rupture. Assess neurovascular status. The patient is usually reluctant to move hand, but overall function should be assessed by asking the patient to make a fist.

To assess ulnar collateral ligament stability, adequate analgesia must be given – Entonox is useful or occasionally local anaesthetic may be inserted. Test ligament integrity by stabilizing the patient's thumb with your middle and index finger over the first metacarpal, and, with the other index finger, gently push on the ulnar aspect of the thumb. Always compare with the other side. Occasionally, stress test views are taken, but this is often too painful in the acute phase.

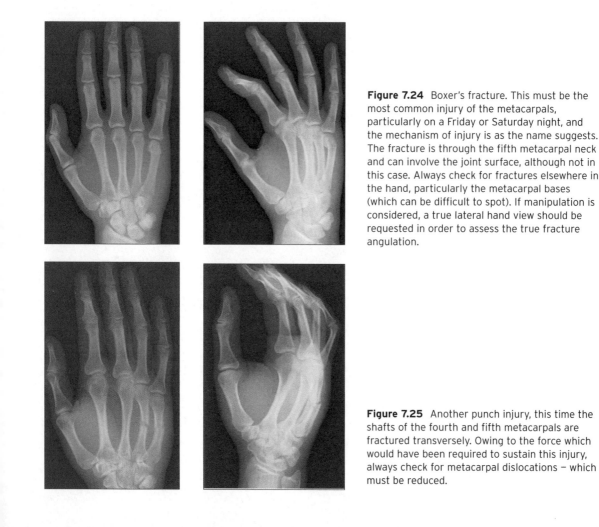

Figure 7.24 Boxer's fracture. This must be the most common injury of the metacarpals, particularly on a Friday or Saturday night, and the mechanism of injury is as the name suggests. The fracture is through the fifth metacarpal neck and can involve the joint surface, although not in this case. Always check for fractures elsewhere in the hand, particularly the metacarpal bases (which can be difficult to spot). If manipulation is considered, a true lateral hand view should be requested in order to assess the true fracture angulation.

Figure 7.25 Another punch injury, this time the shafts of the fourth and fifth metacarpals are fractured transversely. Owing to the force which would have been required to sustain this injury, always check for metacarpal dislocations – which must be reduced.

Figure 7.26 This is an angulated fracture of the fifth metacarpal shaft that has healed with residual angulation. This has caused a shortening of the metacarpal.

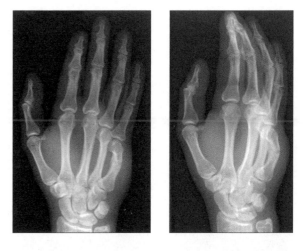

Figure 7.27 Yet another punch injury, this time in a juvenile, resulting in a torus fracture of the metaphysis of the second metacarpal. This is an obvious fracture, but some juvenile boxer's fractures can be easily missed (probably owing to the proximity of the irregular epiphyseal plate).

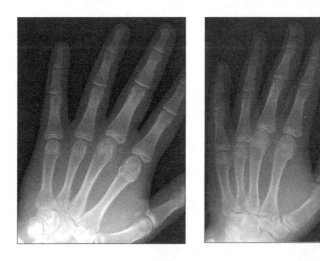

Figure 7.28 It is much harder to spot a small fracture if the area of interest is obscured by other superimposing bony structures, as the eye is not immediately drawn to the abnormality. In this case, there is a small 'corner' or 'chip' fracture at the base of the first metacarpal, but the base of the second metacarpal and the trapezium superimposes this region. Note that this is an intra-articular fracture but not a Bennett's fracture, as it does not cross enough of the metacarpal to render it unstable.

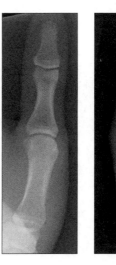
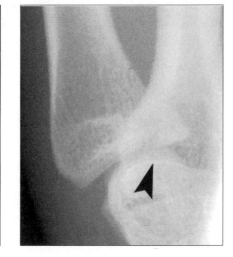

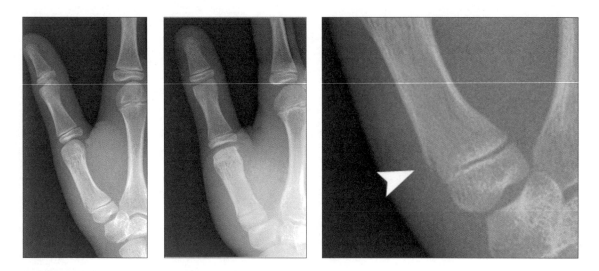

Figure 7.29 Again, a tricky fracture to spot, particularly as the lateral view is poorly positioned resulting in an oblique projection. See detail view below. This fracture communicates with the epiphyseal plate and is therefore a Salter and Harris type II fracture.

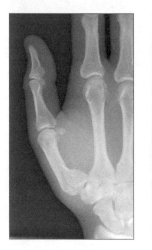 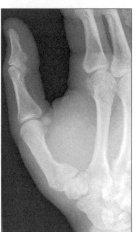

Figure 7.30 A comminuted and slightly displaced fracture of the base of the first metacarpal. This is known as a Bennett's fracture. Owing to the instability of this injury, surgical intervention is normally required.

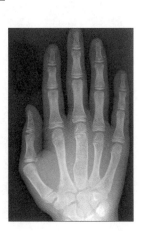 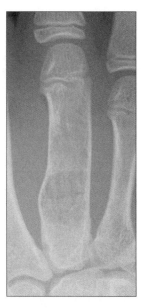

Figure 7.31 This is a pathological fracture of the third metacarpal of a young teenager. The metacarpal has enlarged (*expansile* lesion) and the cortex has thinned, rendering the bone weaker and more vulnerable to mechanical damage. This lesion is an *enchondroma* and is not uncommon. Multiple enchondromata are occasionally seen. This is known as Ollier's disease.

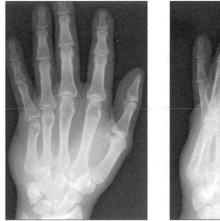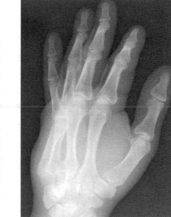

Figure 7.32 There is gross soft-tissue swelling seen here associated with the fifth metacarpal shaft. The DP oblique view (left) demonstrates an abnormal alignment of the fifth metacarpal. In fact, this is dislocated from the normal articulations at the base with the hamate and base of the fourth metacarpal.

Figure 7.33 A useful tool for assessing whether there is a dislocation in the metacarpals. Draw a line (or lay a ruler on the film) joining the middle of the articular surfaces of the fourth and fifth metacarpals on the DP view. Now project this line along to the third metacarpal (as above). It should intersect with the articular surface, as it clearly does in this case. It may also just miss and still be normal owing to a normal variation of metacarpal length. If it clearly misses the head of the third metacarpal and, instead, intersects with the proximal phalanx, look again for a dislocation at the metacarpal bases.

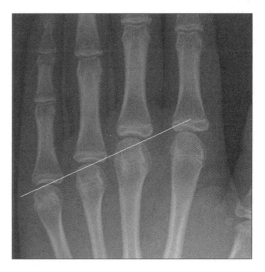

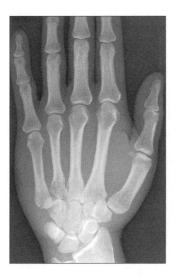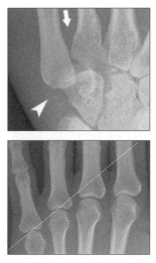

Figure 7.34 In this case, the alignment of the fourth and fifth metacarpals does not intersect with the head of the third metacarpal but crosses the proximal phalanx. There is no fracture, but the base of the fifth metacarpal has dislocated and slipped inferiorly causing the line to 'tip' and miss the third metacarpal head. This is not foolproof, particularly if the metacarpals have been previously fractured, but it is a useful diagnostic tool. This dislocation was missed on two separate occasions, but, by applying this rule (below right), the abnormality becomes apparent. Note that the fifth metacarpal (below left) no longer articulates with the fourth metacarpal base (arrow) or the hamate (arrowhead). Now look back at the dislocation in Figure 7.32 and see if this rule works.

Treatment

Note degree if angulated. Slight to moderate angulation is treated by neighbour strapping and elevation for approximately three to four weeks. Soft-tissue swelling can be severe in these types of injury. Marked angulation (> 45°) needs reduction and occasionally may require open reduction and internal fixation.

Dislocations at the carpo-metacarpal joints (2–5) are rare and easily missed – scrutinize the radiograph for normal alignment.

Bennett's fracture/dislocation should be reduced by an experienced clinician as it is very difficult to maintain the reduction. Occasionally, open reduction and internal fixation is required. Undisplaced fractures (without dislocation) of the first metacarpal are treated in a plaster spica, but angulated fractures must be reduced and/or require internal fixation.

X-rays are taken for avulsion fractures in ulnar collateral ligament rupture. If there is a significant displacement or rotation, the patient needs surgical repair, otherwise, the thumb is immobilized for six weeks.

Chapter 8

The knee joint and distal femur

Review of core anatomy

The knee joint is not only the largest but also the major weight-bearing joint in the body and is entirely dependent on ligaments and muscles for stability and power.

The articular surface of the knee is made up (see Figure 8.3) of the condyles of the femur and the flat tibial plateau, which has two tibial spines in the centre, serving as attachments for the cruciate ligaments. Lying on the tibial plateau are two C-shaped cartilage structures called the menisci, which act as shock absorbers and are joined anteriorly by a transverse ligament preventing them from separating during movements.

The posterior aspect of the lower leg consists mainly of muscles, with the gastrocnemius muscle forming most of the calf. A sesamoid bean-shaped bone, known as the *fabella*, is commonly found inside the lateral head (close to its proximal attachment). This is often visible on the lateral radiograph (see Figure 8.3).

The knee is further stabilized on the sides by the lateral and medial collateral ligaments. The medial collateral ligament is the strongest and connects the femur with the tibia on the medial side, where a deeper layer also joins the medial meniscus. The fibula plays no major role in the knee joint but serves as an attachment for the lateral collateral ligament.

The front of the knee is covered by the patella, which is a sesamoid bone lying within the tendon of the quadriceps. The extensor apparatus of the knee comes from the quadriceps, patella and patellar tendon.

Clinical examination

The mechanism of injury will help guide you towards the structures that may be injured. Remember that the knee is most vulnerable when flexed. A kick to the side of the flexed knee puts it into forced valgus, straining the medial collateral ligament and, should the force be sufficient, additional damage to the meniscus and anterior cruciate ligament (the so-called 'unhappy triad') occurs. A history of clicking, locking or giving way can indicate a meniscal injury.

Look

Observe for swelling and note if the onset was sudden or gradual. Sudden onset is most likely caused by bleeding (haemarthrosis), which may need draining (see Figure 8.13). Localized, soft swelling anterior to the patella that is red and hot to touch is likely to be inflammation of the patella bursae (bursitis). Note any loss of contour from the extensor mechanism. Rupture of the quadriceps tendon is a clinical diagnosis with the history providing the best diagnostic clue (likely mechanism is injury to the knee in full extension). A palpable gap between the tendon and the patella can be felt; although in the acute knee this can be difficult to detect, owing to swelling.

Observe the patient's gait. Is he or she avoiding fully straightening the knee? If so, it must be ascertained whether this is caused by pain, effusion, muscle spasm or a mechanical block within the knee joint (e.g. the presence of a loose foreign body). Observe for any wounds.

Feel

The palpation should start with the knee in full extension and then be repeated in a flexed position to isolate tenderness over joint line. Routinely palpate the:

joint line
femoral condyles
head of the fibula
tibial plateau and tuberosity
patella
ligament insertions

Feel the skin (using the back of your hand) for temperature and compare with the other side. Note any effusions and check the neurovascular status of the ankle/foot for integrity.

Move

As a hinge-type synovial joint, the knee joint allows flexion/extension and is prevented from moving sideways by the collateral ligaments and anteriorly/posteriorly by the cruciate ligaments (see Figure 8.1). A small degree of rotation is also possible when the knee is flexed. These must be tested for laxity. In addition, the menisci should be tested. It is, however, outside the scope of this book to explain the tests used in details, and only a brief review is discussed here. For a fuller explanation and excellent illustrations, we particularly recommend Purcell's (2003) textbook.

Movements should always start with assessing the patient's weight-bearing ability.

Extension: If a patient is capable of a straight-leg raise, the extensor mechanism is intact. However, in the acutely injured knee, extension can be limited by pain, effusion, haemarthrosis and muscle spasm. This must be overcome to assess extension and differentiate from a true locked knee, which is due to a mechanical block, e.g. from a torn meniscus.

Flexion: Observe the degree of flexion and any pain experienced.

Medial and lateral collateral ligament tests are undertaken to observe for pain (elicited in sprains) or laxity (seen in complete rupture).

Draw test: A unique feature of the knee is the appearance of two strong ligaments within the joint known as the anterior and posterior cruciate ligaments (see Figure 8.1). The main function of the posterior cruciate ligament is to prevent the femur moving excessively towards the tibia, e.g. when weight-bearing on a flexed knee. The anterior cruciate ligament prevents slipping of the tibia backward during extension, e.g. when kicking a ball with a straight leg. Ability to pull or push the tibia forward or backward respectively confirms a rupture of either the anterior or posterior cruciate ligament.

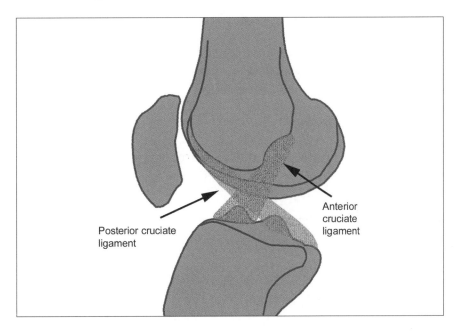

Figure 8.1 Cruciate ligaments. The posterior cruciate ligament prevents forward movement of the femur and the anterior cruciate prevents posterior movement.

Posterior cruciate ligament

Anterior cruciate ligament

Damage to the meniscus is difficult to assess in the acutely injured knee. The history (e.g. locking of knee before end point of flexion or extension) and the presence of a haemarthrosis is the best clue. *McMurray's* or the *grind* tests are used to confirm your suspicion.

Use of radiography in acute knee injuries

Two sets of clinical decision rules have been developed (the Ottawa and the Pittsburgh knee rules) to guide the clinician in their decision as to whether to X-ray or not. Only one study has compared the two sets of rules and found both to have equal sensitivity but found the Pittsburgh rule to be more specific (Seaberg and Jackson, 1994). While both rules have been validated in other settings than the authors' departments, the published evidence for their use is not overwhelming, and the rules should be used with some caution until further research is available. They are, however, useful as a supplement to aid the decision-making process:

Ottawa knee rule (acutely injured knees only)

X-ray if one or more findings are present (Steill et al., 1997):

- age 55 or over
- tenderness at fibula head
- isolated tenderness of the patella
- inability to flex knee to 90°
- inability to weigh-bear* (four steps) both immediately and in the department

Pittsburgh knee rules

In the patient with a history of a fall or blunt trauma, X-ray if one finding is present (Seaberg and Jackson, 1994):

- age < 12 or > 50 or
- inability to walk four weight-bearing steps* in the department

---

* In the Ottawa knee rules, the inability to weight-bear is the inability to transfer weight twice onto the affected leg regardless of limp, whereas the Pittsburgh rule is fully weight-bearing with no limp (Adams, 2004).

Standard projections

AP
lateral

Additional projections

skyline
tunnel
notch

X-ray positioning

In the case of a patient with a fracture or soft-tissue injury, positioning can be difficult. Ideally, the patient will sit on the X-ray table with the knee fully extended and have the two standard views taken. When the reason for requesting an X-ray is acute trauma, the lateral view should always be taken with a horizontal beam to demonstrate fluid levels within the joint capsule; this is explained more fully later in this chapter. Occasionally, patients will find it impossible to fully extend the knee due to injury or loose body causing a 'locked' knee; so the radiographer needs to be sympathetic and obtain the best views possible. The X-ray beam is directed towards a point just below the apex

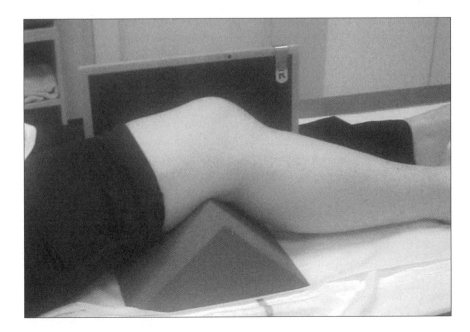

Figure 8.2 In this photograph, the patient is positioned for a horizontal beam lateral of the right knee. The knee is flexed and rested on a foam pad with the X-ray beam parallel to the floor in order to demonstrate a fluid level within the joint capsule. The AP view is taken with the knee extended and directly on the cassette, and the X-ray beam is vertical.

of the patella, which should give a good view of the tibial plateau on the AP view. Both views should include the distal third of the femur and the proximal third of the tibia and fibula. The patella should be central on the film in the AP view, and the femoral condyles should overlap as completely as possible on the lateral view. It is important to demonstrate the soft tissues around the joint well, and for this reason any trousers should be pulled up well above the knee or removed; tight-fitting trousers scrunched up just above the patella cause artefact and obscure the soft tissues.

Radiographic interpretation

Interpretation of the knee views is no more difficult than any other anatomical region. As in all radiographic interpretation, developing a systematic approach to the images will yield dividends rather than staring at an image and hoping that an abnormality will jump out of the film.

For the AP view (see Figure 8.3), trace the cortex of the component bones, including the patella. Pay particular attention to the tibial plateau including the tibial spines for a possible avulsion fracture. Note that in older patients with degenerative changes present the tibial spines can appear markedly 'spiky'. The tibio-femoral joint space should be even; look carefully for any signs of depression that could indicate a subtle tibial plateau fracture. Again, in the older patient narrowing of this joint space, and in particular the medial aspect, can occur. Orthopaedic requests for knee X-ray commonly stipulate that the AP view should be taken with the patient standing – weight-bearing – in order to assess the joint space more accurately. Avulsion fractures of the tibial or femoral margins are also possible. Always check the neck of fibula – this is a fairly common site for missed fractures. Patellar fractures on the AP film can be difficult to spot due to the complete superimposition of the patella over the distal femur.

The lateral view of the knee, either turned as in Figure 8.3 or with a horizontal beam, is interpreted in a similar way. Check the cortex of all the bones first. It is not uncommon to see a second sesamoid bone, the fabella, which lies posterior to the distal femur and occurs in roughly 5%–10% of the population. Trace both femoral condyles; they should overlap, although never completely as the one farthest from the film will be magnified slightly. Check the patella for transverse fractures, which may not show on the AP view.

The suprapatellar pouch is a part of the joint capsule that lies superior to the patella. It is not normally seen except when, owing to injury or infection, there is a joint effusion and the pouch becomes distended

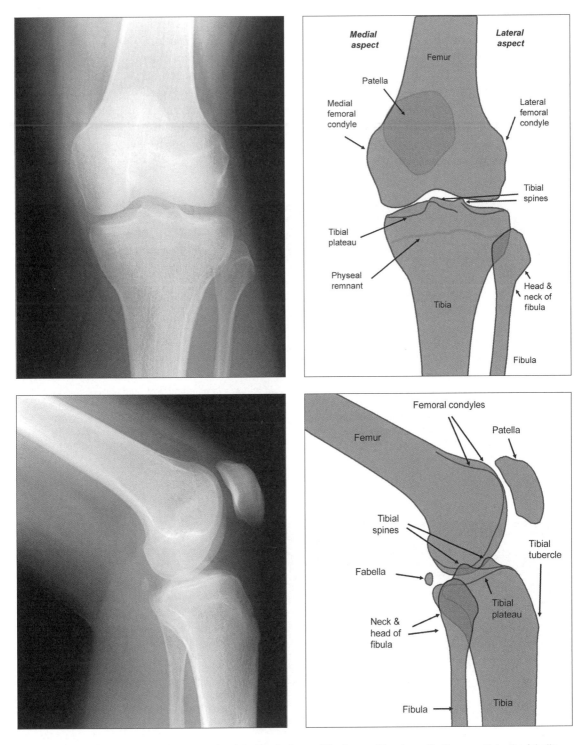

Figure 8.3 Normal AP (top) and turned lateral (bottom) views of the knee with schematic diagram. Note the fabella seen on the lateral view just posterior to the femoral condyles, which is a normal variant.

with fluid. A large joint effusion is seen in Figure 8.4. If there is a fracture within the confines of the joint capsule, fat from the medullary cavity leaks into the capsule. The fat, being less dense than blood or synovial fluid, will float to the highest point of the joint capsule and form a fat/fluid interface with a darker plane above the denser blood beneath. This phenomenon is known as a lipohaemarthrosis and is only seen if the X-ray beam passes tangentially across the joint and the fluid level, thus all knee X-rays done post-trauma should be with a horizontal beam to demonstrate this.

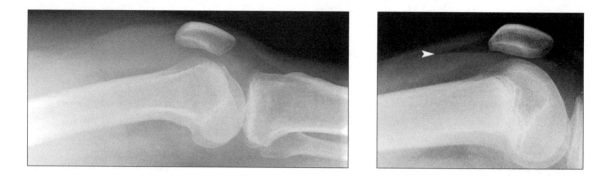

Figure 8.4 Joint effusion and lipohaemarthrosis. In the left-hand figure, a large amount of fluid has collected within the joint capsule and been forced up into the suprapatellar pouch. This has resulted in the bulbous grey region seen superior to the patella, and this has tipped the patella anteriorly and inferiorly In the right-hand figure, a horizontal line (white arrowhead) is seen in the pouch separating a region of synovial fluid and blood (below) from a layer of fat (above) that has leaked from a fracture site. Even if a fracture line is not visible, the presence of a lipohaemarthrosis is indicative of an occult (unseen) fracture.

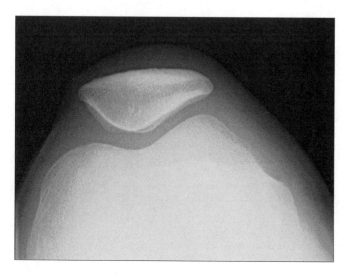

Figure 8.5 Normal skyline view. This is obtained with the patient sitting up and holding the cassette against the distal femur, the knee is flexed to about 60° and the X-ray beam is directed horizontally to pass through the patello-femoral joint. It can be useful if a longitudinal patellar fracture is suspected but is contra-indicated in the case of a possible transverse fracture as the fracture fragments could be further separated. Note that the patella sits in the groove between the femoral condyles with an even joint space.

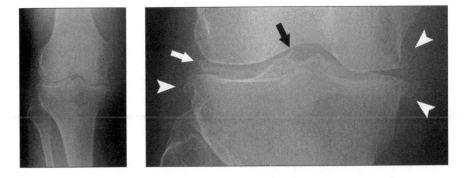

Figure 8.6 Degenerative changes in the knee joint. In this example, of the right knee of a 77-year-old woman, there are several changes due to degenerative disease that should not be confused with an acute injury. Marginal osteophytosis is present; in other words, the bone has formed a lip – white arrowheads, detail view (below). There is chondrocalcinosis of the meniscal cartilage, which is principally due to mineral deposits within the cartilage – white arrow, detail view (below), and there is a spiking of the tibial spine – black arrow, detail view (below). Additionally, the medial joint compartment is slightly narrowed, although this is only minimal in this case.

As well as checking for mechanical trauma such as fractures and dislocations, always check the texture of the bone for abnormalities. In particular, the femoral condyles are susceptible to disruption to the cartilage lining the joint surface, which can cause a section of bone to detach – known as an osteochondral fracture. A more chronic effect is osteochondritis. So look for any disruption to the normal even texture of the trabecular pattern.

Ligamentous injuries

As the knee relies on ligaments for stability, the long-term consequences of severe ligamentous injuries are serious. However, as ligaments do not show up on a radiograph it is outside the scope of this book to discuss these in detail. The only exception is that of a complete ligament rupture in which an avulsion fracture is sustained:

Cruciate ligament rupture: plain X-ray will show avulsion of one or both of the tibial spines (see Figure 8.23)

Medial collateral ligament: often associated with anterior cruciate ligament tear, but isolated tears can also occur. Flake fractures can be seen at the femoral attachment and lead to new bone formation, a condition known as Pelligrini-Steida disease (see Figure 8.16).

Distal femoral fractures

We have not included hip or femoral shaft fractures in this text as they cannot be considered minor injuries. However, fractures of the distal femur may be encountered in an MIU and are therefore included here.

Supracondylar fractures in adults are usually caused by forced flexion or hyperextension and tend to rotate into posterior angulation, owing to the pull of the gastrocnemius muscle. In children, supracondylar fractures tend to lead to a slipped lower femoral epiphysis with minimal displacement. The knee will look swollen and often deformed. The patient is in severe pain, and it is often difficult to fully palpate all structures of the knee. The distal neurovascular integrity must be assessed. The patient will be non-weight-bearing and unable to straight-leg raise. It will usually be far too painful to attempt to assess any ligaments.

All distal femur and condylar fractures are referred to orthopaedics.

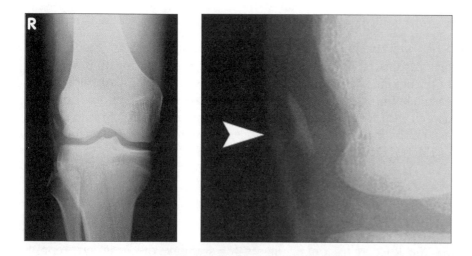

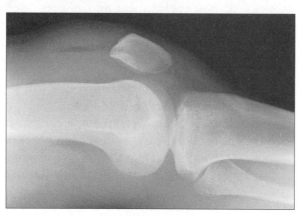

Figure 8.7 Femoral avulsion fracture. A fragment of bone is seen avulsed from the lateral aspect of the distal femur – AP view (top left) and detail view (top right) as a result of a twisting injury. A lipohaemarthrosis is present on the lateral view (bottom), but the fracture itself cannot be reliably seen owing to the superimposition of bony structures.

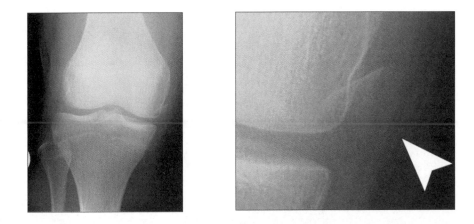

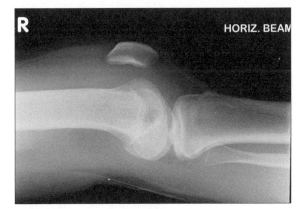

Figure 8.8 Another avulsion fracture from the distal femur, this one from the medial aspect. Note that the fragment is seen to be trabeculated and corticated along one edge. Again, the lateral view (bottom) demonstrates an effusion with elevation of the patella due to the bulkiness of the suprapatellar pouch.

Figure 8.9 This is a spiral fracture of the distal femur, which is shown on both views and can be seen to extend into the joint. This is a severe injury resulting from an RTA as a pedestrian.

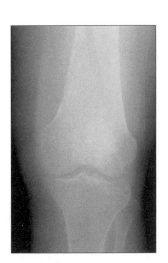

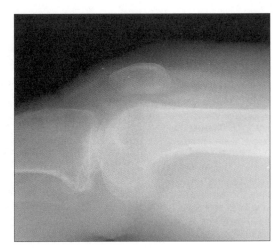

Figure 8.10 This is an intercondylar fracture of the distal femur that extends into the joint. There is joint effusion but no lipohaemarthrosis is seen. Both injuries need orthopaedic referral.

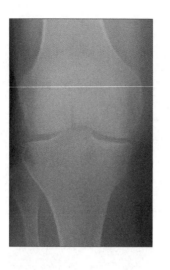
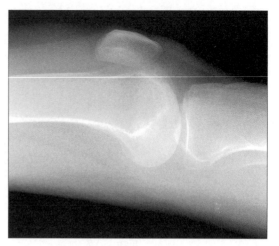

Figure 8.11 A subtle fracture of the medial femoral condyle. When there is degenerative change, very careful scrutiny of the cortex is required as fractures tend to be more easily overlooked. The lateral view (right) is distorted as the patient was in great pain and the leg could not be moved for optimum positioning.

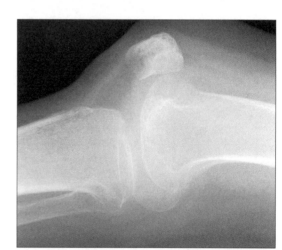

Figure 8.12 This is a greenstick fracture of the distal femur. There is a shift of the lateral aspect of the metaphysis with respect to the epiphysis. The fracture line extends from the buckle seen at the medial side of the shaft to the lateral aspect of the physeal line. This would be classified as a Salter and Harris type II fracture.

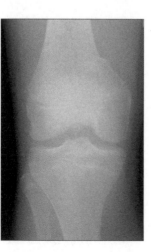
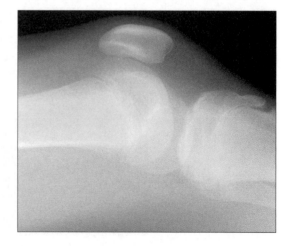

Treatment

A haemarthrosis always indicates a severe injury and should be drained as blood within the knee acts as glue that usually clots causing adhesions within the joint, restricting movements. Unclotted blood causes severe synovitis that can take weeks to heal (Dandy and Edwards, 2003). The knee is aspirated (see Figure 8.13) and the blood examined for fat globules, as fat is only ever present within the knee joint from a fracture.

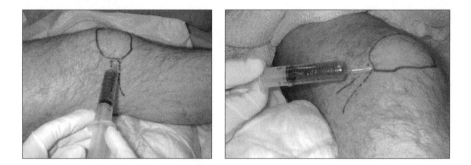

Figure 8.13 Knee aspiration. Lay the patient on a couch with the knee in approximately 30° flexion. It is often easier to find the joint space with the knee flexed. In fact, the presence of a large haematoma may actually prevent the knee from fully extending. The knee should be cleaned with an iodine/antiseptic solution and sterile gloves worn. Install a small amount of local anaesthetic to the subcutaneous tissue. Using a large-bore needle (approximately 18 gauge) attached to a large syringe (an intravenous cannula with a three-way tap at the end can also be used), insert it at the lateral or medial margin of the patella. Aspirate blood – it should be easy to drain if present.

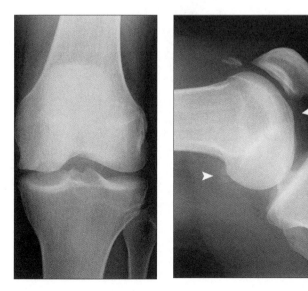

Figure 8.14 Osteochondral fracture. Look at the articular surface of the medial femoral condyle on the AP view (left): there is an elliptical-shaped lucency that represents an osteochondral fracture at this point. A portion of the articular bony surface has fractured away along with the cartilaginous lining of the bone surface leaving the lucent appearance. The lateral view (right) shows one loose fragment in the suprapatellar pouch and two smaller fragments just posterior to the femoral condyles (arrowhead). The bony defect is seen as an irregularity just below the patella (arrow). Fractures involving only the cartilage also occur but, of course, will be invisible on conventional radiographs. In chondral or osteochondral fractures, further imaging is required by arthrography, MRI or possibly CT to evaluate the extent of the injury. The mechanism of injury is usually twisting, shearing or direct impact (e.g. a skiing accident).

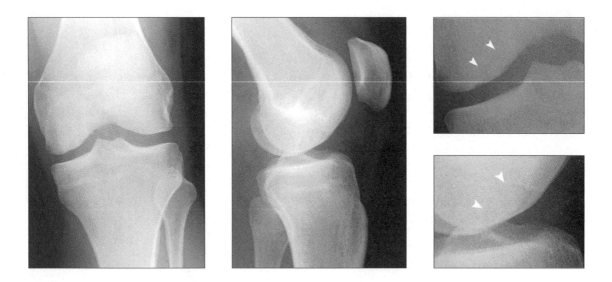

Figure 8.15 Osteochondritis dissicans in the medial femoral condyle. Compare these images with the previous examination of an osteochondral fracture (white arrowheads on both detail views). The position and appearance are similar, but osteochondritis dissicans is generally considered to be a chronic process as a result of repeated relatively low-grade trauma rather than a single event, as in acute osteochondral fracture (Greenspan, 2000). The appearance tends to be more irregular, although with unchecked progression ultimately a bony fragment may become isolated and dislodged and migrate within the joint capsule, where it can block extension (a true 'locked' knee). Again, further imaging is required to evaluate the extent of joint damage as the soft-tissue injury cannot be seen on the plain films. Arthrography, arthroscopy, CT or MRI can be used to assess the injury more fully.

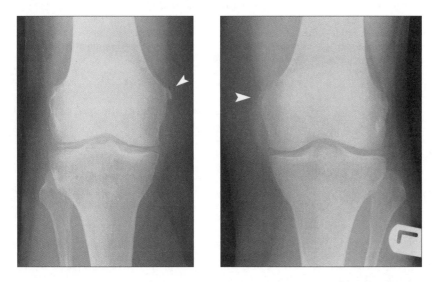

Figure 8.16 Pelligrini-Steida lesions. The Pelligrini-Steida lesion is seen as a partial calcification of the medial collateral ligament at its insertion point on the medial femoral condyle (Greenspan, 2000). Two examples are presented here from different patients (white arrowheads). It occurs following a tear to the medial collateral ligament and is a chronic rather than an acute finding. Thus, this appearance is indicative of injury from some time in the past. Note that the patient on the left also has chondrocalcinosis of the menisci.

Injuries to the patella and the extensor mechanism

The mechanism of injury is usually caused by a direct trauma to the patella or a violent contraction of the quadriceps. If the patella dislocates, it usually does so laterally. It is common in adolescent girls with lax ligaments and often reduces itself spontaneously. The knee looks swollen with a haemarthrosis, which is visible on the radiograph. A rupture of the quadriceps leads to more-generalized swelling, with a 'high'-riding patella lying more proximally. Bruising and generalized swelling is seen in a fractured patella. There will be some localized tenderness over the fracture site and the insertion point of the patella and quadriceps tendons, which may also avulse. A palpable gap between the tendon and the patella may be felt when the quadriceps has ruptured, but is often obscured in the acute phase due to diffuse swelling. The patient will be unable to fully weight-bear or extend the knee. If the extensor mechanism is impaired, the patient will not be able to straight-leg raise.

When reviewing radiographs, patellar fractures must be distinguished from a bipartite or tripartite patella (see Figure 8.18).

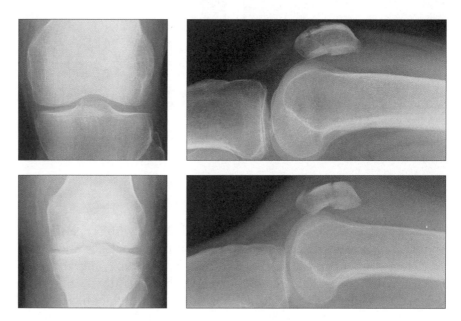

Figure 8.17 Patellar fractures. Two examples of patellar fractures are shown above. Both are comminuted and both have a joint effusion well shown on the lateral view. The fractures are seen on both views but are more easily detected on the lateral views (right, top and bottom) as there is no superimposition of bone structures. If a transverse fracture of the patella is suspected, skyline views should not be requested as the knee flexion necessary to achieve the image will potentially separate the fragments further. A common normal variant is a bipartite patella, which is where the patella forms from two (or more) separate ossification centres that do not necessarily unite, even in adulthood. Figure 8.18 (next page) shows two examples of bipartite patellae (left) and two tripartite patellae (right). The smaller components are usually seen in the upper lateral region. These appearances should not be confused with a patellar fracture.

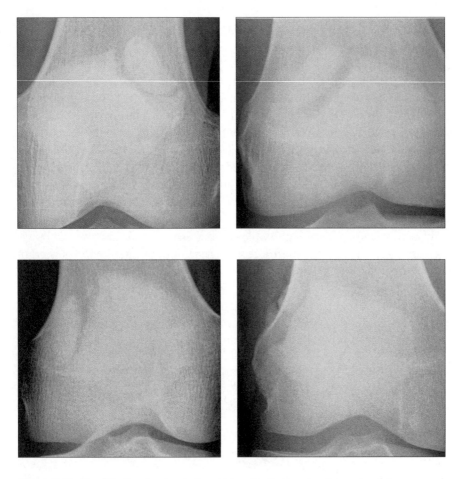

Figure 8.18 Bipartite (top two images) and tripartite (bottom two images) patellae.

Treatment

Undisplaced patellar fractures are treated in a cylinder plaster (or splint) for six weeks. Displaced or comminuted fractures should be discussed with orthopaedics, as internal fixation may be required. Occasionally, the patella is removed. Any haemarthrosis should be drained to reduce pain and any dislocations should be reduced. First, dislocations are treated with a plaster or a splint but recurrent dislocations are treated supportively with physiotherapy. Avulsion fractures to the tibial tubercle in adults are treated in a cylinder plaster or occasionally internally fixated if there is a marked displacement. In children, internal fixation is avoided if at all possible to prevent premature epiphyseal fusion.

Fractures of the tibial plateau

The mechanism of injury is usually due to a violent blow to the lateral side of the knee stressing the medial aspect, tearing the medial collateral ligament and fracturing the lateral aspect of the tibial plateau. A haemarthrosis may be present together with bruising, but there is rarely any deformity of note. There is some tenderness over the tibial plateau and generalized pain, and the patient is usually unable to weight-bear and any full assessment of ligaments may be too painful to undertake.

All tibial plateau fractures are referred to orthopaedics.

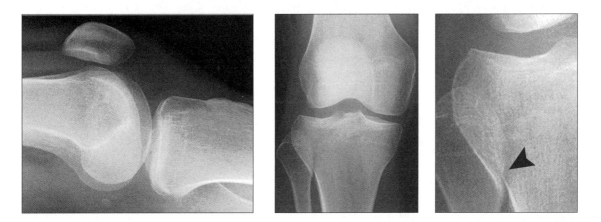

Figure 8.19 Tibial plateau fracture (I). This is a relatively undisplaced fracture of the lateral tibial plateau. On the AP view (bottom left), the main cortical break happens to coincide with the medial fibula neck outline – black arrowhead on detail view (bottom right), which results in a fracture that isn't quite as obvious as it is serious. Look at the tibial plateau itself, however, and it does tip upwards at its lateral aspect, and there is a misalignment of the lateral femoral condyle with the lateral aspect of the tibia. The lateral view (top) has no discernible fracture line; however, there is a prominent lipohaemarthrosis that indicates the presence of a fracture within the joint capsule. This is shown as the fat/blood interface with the fat layer floating on the blood and resulting in the patella tipping forward somewhat. A CT scan would demonstrate the extent of the injury more fully.

Figure 8.20 Tibial plateau fracture (II). The fracture line on the AP view (left) is more obvious than the example in Figure 8.19. The lipohaemarthrosis is present on the lateral view (right) as are fracture lines. However, the true extent of the injury is only demonstrated with a CT scan of the knee (Figure 8.21) with coronal reconstructions – in other words, 'slices' – through the knee from front to back.

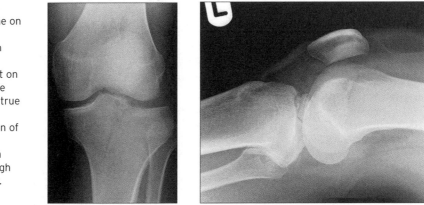

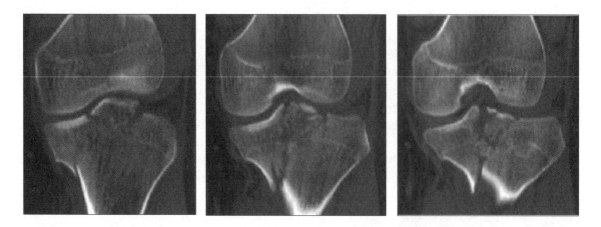

Figure 8.21 CT slices that progress posteriorly through the joint show the fragmentation and instability of the fracture. CT is a very useful tool for the orthopaedic surgeon to plan the surgery required. Note again the misalignment of the lateral aspects of the femur and tibia, indicating a spreading of the tibial plateau.

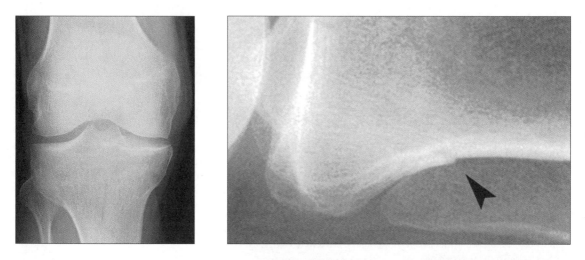

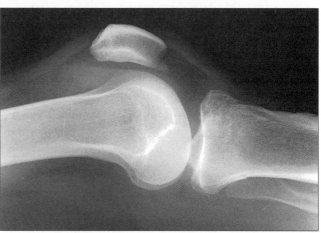

Figure 8.22 Tibial plateau fracture (III). This fracture is much more subtle – see detail view (top right) – than either of the previous examples and demonstrates the need for a very careful inspection of all aspects of both views. There is no clear fracture line or widening of the joint spaces on the AP view (top left) to indicate a depression of the tibial plateau; but on the lateral view (bottom) a subtle step in the cortex posteriorly is seen together with a fairly indistinct fracture line passing superiorly and anteriorly into the joint. A lipohaemarthrosis is present with the resultant elevation of the patella. Probably an easy fracture to miss except that the presence of the lipohaemarthrosis would make that inexcusable.

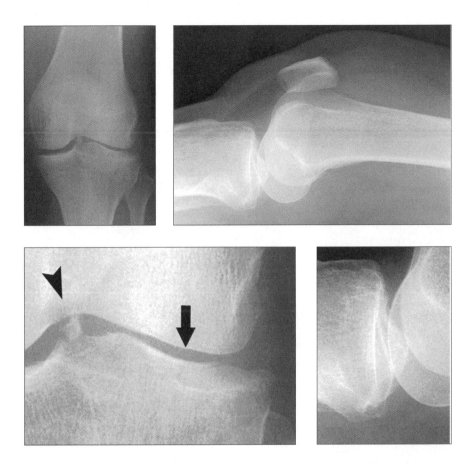

Figure 8.23 Tibial plateau fracture (IV). There is an avulsion-type fracture of the tibial spine, which is easily seen (black arrowhead), but there is also a very slightly depressed fracture of the lateral tibial plateau which is not quite so obvious (black arrow). A useful tip in identifying tibial plateau fractures is to draw normal alignment lines (see Figure 8.24). The tibial plateau fracture is not apparent on the lateral view but, again, the lipohaemarthrosis is present and provides the vital clue. This example shows how more than one fracture can be present on the same examination and, in this case, how this increases the seriousness of the injury greatly. Do not fall into the trap of 'search satisfaction' when one abnormality is found; continue to scrutinize the films until you have excluded further injury.

Figure 8.24 Draw a line laterally against the femur down to the tibia. In the normal knee, no more than a maximum of 5 mm of the tibia should lie outside the line. If the articular surface of the tibia is projecting more than 5 mm beyond the line, a tibial plateau fracture should be suspected. Try to apply this principle to Figure 8.25 and then to Figure 8.19.

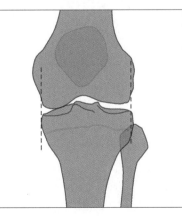
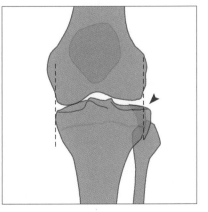

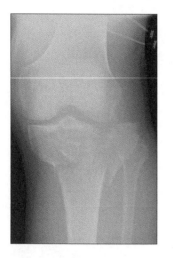

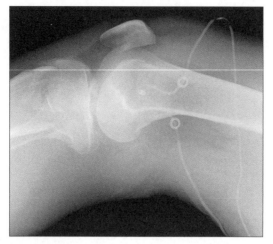

Figure 8.25 Tibial plateau fracture (V). This examination demonstrates just how severe these fractures can be. Note the degree of displacement of the lateral view (right) of the tibial plateau and how the fibula has been displaced laterally also.

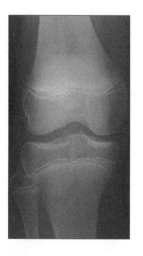

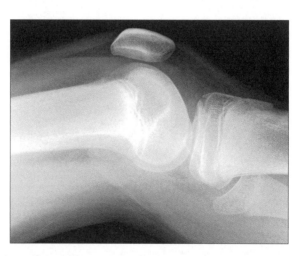

Figure 8.26 Tibial plateau fracture (VI). This is a fracture through the middle of the epiphysis in a young male patient following an RTA. The fracture line extends to the growth plate and has also damaged the tibial spine. This would be classified as a Salter and Harris type III fracture. The lipohaemarthrosis is a clear indicator of bony injury.

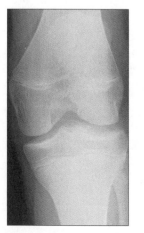

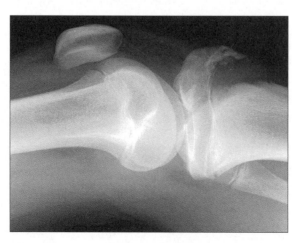

Figure 8.27 A truly startling injury, the tibial tubercle and the anterior half of the epiphysis have been wrenched superiorly. Note the migration of the patella away from the joint. The AP view (left) is surprisingly normal. Surgical intervention would be required here to reduce and stabilize the fracture.

Figure 8.28 Segond fracture. This is another avulsion fracture, this time of the lateral aspect of the proximal tibia just below the tibial plateau. Two examples are shown here. The appearance is of a small fragment of bone pulled away from the cortex, which is attached to the lateral capsular ligament. This injury can be associated with a capsular tear, lateral meniscal tear and a tear of the anterior cruciate ligament contributing to joint instability (Greenspan, 2000). Further imaging with arthroscopy or MRI is required to evaluate the extent of the injury. Note that in the example on the right there is a narrowing of the joint space medially and a misalignment of the lateral borders of the femur and tibia (arrowhead).

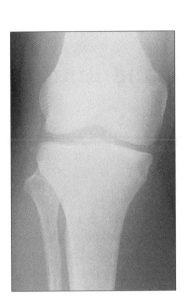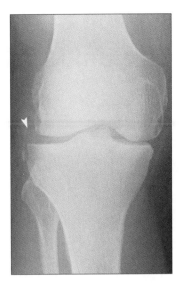

Figure 8.29 Fibular neck/head fracture. This is a fairly common finding and may occur in conjunction with a distal tibial fracture (so-called 'ring of bone' or 'contre-coup' injury). Because these fractures often lie outside the joint's synovial capsule, an effusion is not always present. Occasionally, these can be hard to spot if the tibia is projected over the fibula. Always identify and trace the cortex of both bones individually.

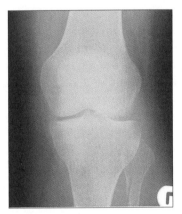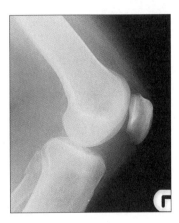

Figure 8.30 A strange-looking film to complete the chapter – this is a bony exostosis or solitary osteochondroma in an adolescent boy. Basically, this is excess bone with a cartilage cap attached to the main shaft by a stalk. Note that the stalk has fractured. This patient was followed up and the lesion was proved to be benign. Findings of this sort on the radiograph must without exception be checked with a consultant radiologist with possible orthopaedic referral to exclude malignancy.

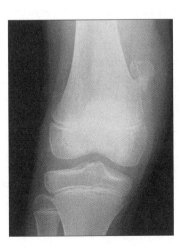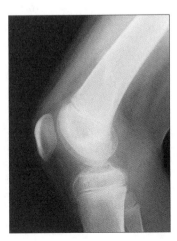

Chapter 9

The ankle joint and hind-foot

Review of core anatomy

The lower leg consists of two long bones: medially, the tibia and, laterally, the fibula. The tibia is the largest and the main weight-bearing bone of the lower leg and is easily palpated anteriorly. At its proximal end, the tibia forms the tibial plateau. A transverse section of the tibia reveals it to be triangular in shape. The fibula bears no weight and forms a head proximally at the knee. The head is palpable, but the shaft of the fibula is not, as it is covered by muscle. The tibia and fibula are joined together by an interosseous membrane and functionally operate as one bone.

The most important aspect of the tibia's and fibula's anatomies is distally where they help form the ankle joint. Distally, both bones project into bony styloid processes, known as the *malleoli*. The tibial end forms the medial malleolus and the fibular end the lateral malleolus, which sits slightly lower than the medial. The malleoli are easily palpated. The inferior surface of the tibia (at times also described as the 'third' malleolus) articulates with the fibula at the distal tibio-fibular joint held strongly together by the anterior and posterior talo-fibular ligaments. The posterior talo-fibular ligament is extremely strong to prevent the foot bones moving up between the tibia and fibula.

Together with the talus and the inferior surface of the tibia, the malleoli form a hinge-type joint. This is often compared to a mortise and tendon joint with the trochlea of the talus being the tendon and the malleoli and the articular surface of the tibia, the mortise. The strong relationship and dependency between the mortise joint, ligaments and the interosseous membrane is described as a syndesmosis.

Although anatomically the talus and the calcaneus are foot bones, they are included in this chapter due to their articulation with and essential function of a normal ankle. The talus sits on the anterior two-thirds of the calcaneus and is shaped like a saddle when viewed dorsally. Anatomically, the talus has a body, neck and a head. The body articulates with the tibia and fibula and the head with the navicular. The neck lies in between. The talus depends on the integrity of the joint for its blood supply, and fractures to the waist of the talus can

Figure 9.1 The talus fits into the mortise joint of the ankle comprising the malleoli, the inferior surface of the tibia and the posterior tibio-fibular ligament.

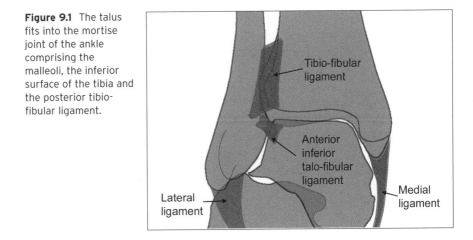

cause avascular necrosis to its proximal end. The calcaneus is the strongest and largest bone in the foot. It has a near-rectangular shape and articulates with the cuboid anteriorly. The calcaneus articulates with the talus at the subtalar (talo-calcaneal) joint, which is a synovial joint between the inferior surface of the body of the talus and the superior surface of the calcaneus, supported by the talo-calcaneal ligaments.

The foot receives its blood supply from the anterior and posterior tibial artery (divisions of the popliteal artery), with further subdivision into several branches, some of which join on the dorsum of the foot to form an arch. The nerve supply to the lower leg is complex but has five terminal branches supplying the ankle and foot. Consequently, the whole of the foot must be thoroughly assessed to ensure that the integrity of all the branches are evaluated.

Clinical examination

Injuries to the ankle and shaft of the tibia and fibula occur mainly as inversion/eversion injuries, although direct trauma can also be responsible. The injuries sustained by this mechanism can range from a minor sprain to a limb-threatening fracture/dislocated ankle, especially if other forces such as rotation or compression are involved. To anticipate the likely damage, it is useful to ask the patient to demonstrate, using the uninjured limb, the exact mechanism of injury.

The tibia and fibula are held together by the interosseous membrane and several ligaments. Like the radius and ulna in the forearm, the net effect is that of a bundle of sticks tied together acting as one. Therefore, there is a high likelihood of injuries to both bones, except when direct trauma has occurred. The onus is on the clinician to positively exclude injury to the other bone, and a thorough clinical examination of the knee and ankle must be undertaken. Any positive findings must be stated on the X-ray request form to ensure both joints are X-rayed if so indicated. Past injuries are noted as patients may present with weak ligaments from repeated injuries.

Look

An examination must include exposure of both legs up to and including the knee. Compare limbs for bruising (may not be present if early presentation) and swelling. Immediate swelling indicates a more severe injury than slow-developing (over a few hours) swelling (Nurse and Rimmer, 2002). Observe for any obvious deformity. A fractured/dislocated ankle (may be known as a Pott's fracture described by Sir Percival Pott in 1769) is a clinical diagnosis and should always be reduced before any X-rays are taken as the limb is under serious neurovascular compromise. The skin may appear critical, i.e. non-blanching and tense if the bone ends are pressed hard against it. Occasionally, bone ends may perforate the skin.

Feel

Starting at the knee, routinely palpate all anatomical structures:

- fibular head
- tibial plateau and shaft of tibia
- medial and lateral malleoli
- base of fifth metatarsal
- mid-foot bones and metatarsals
- posterior tibio-fibular ligament
- anterior talo-fibular ligament
- lateral and medial ligaments

Ensure neurovascular assessment is undertaken by evaluating sensation, pulses and capillary refill in the foot.

Move

The neutral position is when the foot is at a right angle to the leg (Dean and Pegington, 1996). The ankle movements are uniaxial with dorsi- (20°) and plantar- (50°) flexion. When the foot is plantar-flexed, some adduction (inversion – approximately 30°); abduction (eversion – approximately 10°) and rotation are possible (Purcell, 2003).

Assess active movements and undertake passive only if the patient can tolerate these. Resisted movements are reserved until after a fracture has been ruled out on the radiograph. To assess the integrity of the anterior talo-fibular ligament, the anterior draw test is useful, but it is very unreliable if the patient has not been given adequate analgesia. The knee is fully flexed and the ankle is held in 10° plantar-flexion. The examiner places one hand on the leg and pushes backward on it while the examiner's other hand pulls the patient's heel forward under the tibia. If positive, the talus can be moved forward and backward and the Achilles tendon may appear flat (Purcell, 2003; Wardrope and English, 1998).

Assess the patient's weight-bearing abilities and in particular note how long after an injury they lost the ability to walk. Immediate inability to weight-bear after an injury raises the suspicion of a fracture.

Ottawa ankle rules

The Ottawa ankle rules (Steill et al., 1995) are based upon decision-making criteria regarding the need for an X-ray and have been extensively studied and validated. The rules seek to determine if an X-ray is indicated and, if so, whether it should be an ankle or a foot X-ray to be requested, as rarely both are needed.

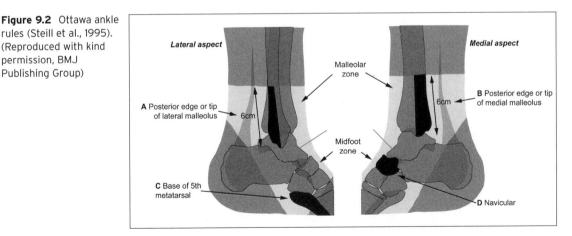

Figure 9.2 Ottawa ankle rules (Steill et al., 1995). (Reproduced with kind permission, BMJ Publishing Group)

An ankle X-ray series is required only if there is any pain in the malleolar zone and any of these findings:

- bone tenderness at A
- bone tenderness at B
- inability to bear weight both immediately and when examined

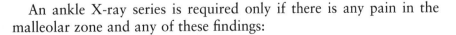

Standard projections

AP and lateral – if a shaft fracture is suspected, the entire length of the tibia and fibula should be included, otherwise the distal third of the tibia and fibula is sufficient for ankle injuries.

Additional projections

os calcis (axial calcaneal)
oblique/mortise

X-ray positioning

The standard views, even with severe injury, are usually straightforward to obtain provided handling of the limb is carried out carefully and sympathetically. The patient sits on the X-ray table with their legs extended and the foot at 90° to the lower leg. For the AP view, the leg is internally rotated approximately 15° from neutral to bring the little toe vertically above the centre of the heel. The X-ray beam is directed to a point midway between the malleoli, and the view should include from the distal third of the tibia and fibula to the talus and navicular. The tarsal bones below the talus are not adequately visualized on the ankle series. Strictly speaking, this is not a true AP view as the leg is internally rotated, but this position demonstrates the mortise joint space well.

Positioning for the lateral view requires the patient to turn towards the affected side so that the lateral malleolus is in contact with the

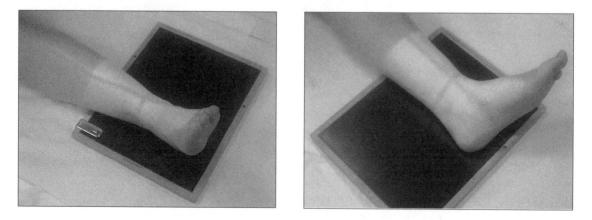

Figure 9.3 X-ray positioning for ankle AP (left) and lateral (right) views.

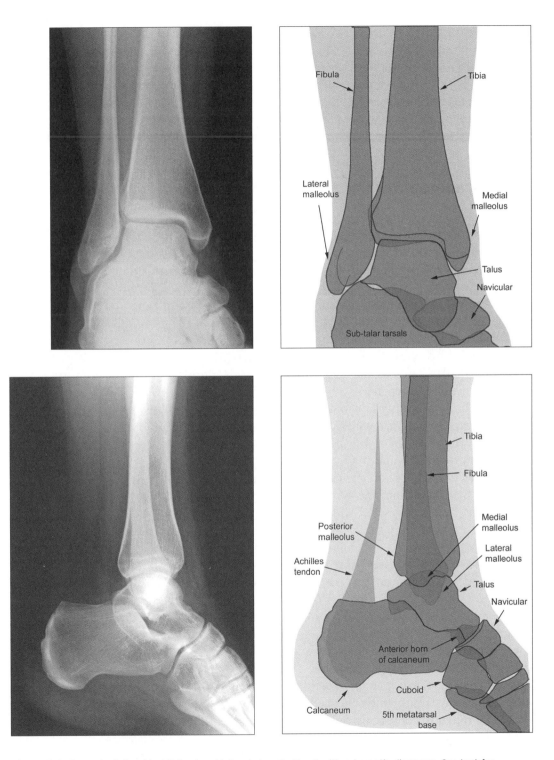

Figure 9.4 Normal adult ankle AP (top) and lateral view (bottom) with schematic diagrams. See text for radiographic interpretation.

film. The little toe should align horizontally with the centre of the heel, this is achieved by rotating the leg about 15° up from the horizontal. This should result in the fibula being superimposed over the tibia and the navicular and base of the fifth metatarsal should be demonstrated on the image. Patients may be imaged with the lower leg immobilized in a box splint, although invariably there will be artefact on the image.

Radiographic interpretation

On both views, trace the cortex of all the bony structures and pay special attention to any overlapping bones. On the AP view, the mortise joint comprising the distal fibula, tibia and talus should have an even joint space all the way round the three sides of the joint with no evidence of any tilting of the articular surface of the talus. Look carefully at the malleoli: undisplaced fractures here are relatively common and can be difficult to spot. Examine the articular surface of the talus looking for any lucencies that might indicate an osteochondral fracture or osteochondritis dissicans (see later in this chapter). In direct trauma, a crack, particularly across the fibular shaft, can be almost invisible so use a magnifier if necessary.

Rather more anatomy is demonstrated on the lateral view as some of the subtarsal bones are well shown. The fibular shaft should be centrally superimposed over the distal tibia. Trace the cortex of both bones right down to each malleolus. An oblique fracture of the distal fibula often only shows on the lateral view, but, because it is superimposed on the distal tibia, the eye may not be immediately drawn to it. On the AP view, it does not show either because it is viewed *en face* rather than tangentially as with the lateral. Look carefully at the dorsum of the talus and the navicular; avulsion fractures are possible here and are occasionally missed. The base of the fifth metatarsal should be visible and is a common site for an avulsion fracture following an inversion injury.

The calcaneus is a site of fracture following a fall from a height. Assess the shape of the bone and the trabecular pattern for subtle fractures. Trace the outline of the cortex right up to the anterior horn – this is a commonly missed fracture. The Achilles tendon shows well against the soft-tissue planes as a black elongated triangular stripe, although X-ray is not routinely used to diagnose Achilles tendon rupture. The diagnosis is usually on clinical signs; although ultrasound is also useful. Look out also in the soft tissues for signs of an effusion that can indicate the severity of trauma – for an example of this see Figure 9.15.

The paediatric ankle

Figure 9.5 Normal juvenile ankle. The same scanning technique is required as for the adult views – check alignments of the epiphyses very carefully as fractures through the growth plates are notoriously missable. The posterior calcaneal apophysis is often very dense as in this example, which is also divided. This is normal and part of the developmental process.

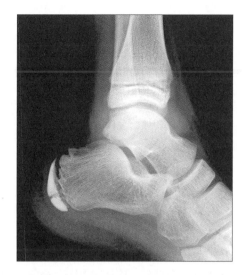

Figure 9.6 Normal variants. There are many accessory bones around the ankle and foot that can sometimes confuse the unwary as they can mimic a fracture. The bony process arising from the posterior aspect of the talus, seen in two examples here (white arrowheads) could be mistaken for a fracture. It is known as an 'os trigonum' when it forms as a secondary ossification centre as in these cases, although the size and degree of separation from the talus does vary. The example in the left-hand image is less distinctly separate than that in the centre.

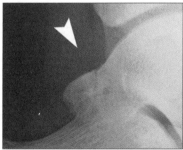

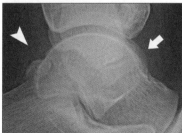

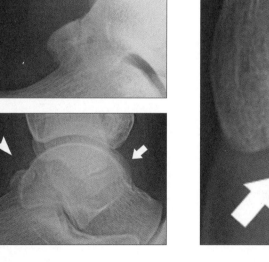

A second variant occasionally seen in the ankle is the separate anterior colliculus, which is one of the two tips of the lateral malleolus (white arrows, bottom left and right-hand images). In this example the appearance, particularly in the lateral view, could be mistaken for a fracture; however, it is rounded with a sclerotic border unlike that of a fracture fragment. Both these examples of normal variants show the need to be aware that they may be encountered and that they are not uncommon. It is very useful to have a copy of Keat (1996) to hand when looking at radiographs – it is a superb reference work presenting the skeletal variants that can mimic fractures and other pathology. In our opinion, anyone using X-rays for diagnosis should have access to a copy.

Distal tibial and fibular fractures

Injuries to the distal tibia and fibula range from sprained ligaments to multiple fractures in a variety of combinations. A simple method to describe/classify ankle fractures that is useful for MIUs is based on using description and the level of the fracture in relation to the mortise. *Always remember there may be an associated fracture proximally of either the tibia or fibula.*

Description

single, isolated fracture to either malleoli
bimalleolar
trimalleolar (the third malleolus being the posterior margin of the
    distal tibia)

Level of fracture

fibular fractures at or above the level of the joint are unstable and
    should be referred
tibial fractures are generally always unstable except for avulsion
    fractures to the medial malleolus.

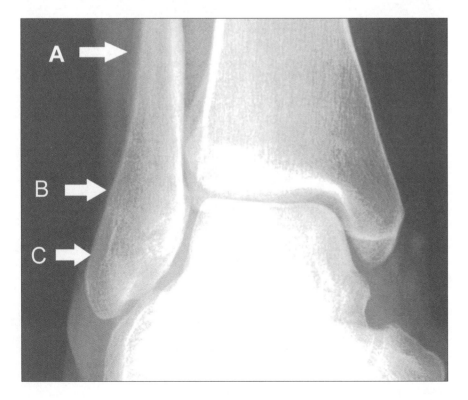

Figure 9.7 Level of injury in relation to the ankle joint. The level of injury is defined according to the position of the fracture as follows: A: above level of joint, B: at level of joint and C: below level of joint.

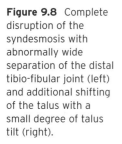

Figure 9.8 Complete disruption of the syndesmosis with abnormally wide separation of the distal tibio-fibular joint (left) and additional shifting of the talus with a small degree of talus tilt (right).

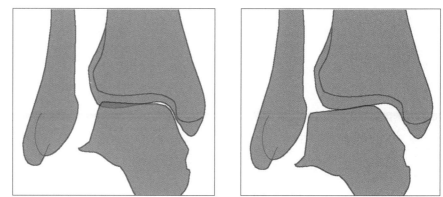

Depending on the severity, there will be localized or diffuse swelling. Deformity may be present. Bruising may not be present if the patient presents early. In ligamentous injuries alone, the tenderness will be localized, although general pain may be felt throughout the ankle. The posterior aspect of the malleoli should be palpated to isolate bone tenderness from ligamentous tenderness. Pulses, sensation and capillary refill must be assessed in the foot. In isolated ligamentous injuries weight-bearing may be possible, as are some movements, with restriction isolated to the affected ligament only. The anterior draw test is useful in detecting a complete rupture of ligaments, but is unreliable if the patient hasn't had adequate analgesia. It should not be undertaken until a fracture has been ruled out. Some patients may be partially weight-bearing with avulsion fracture of the lateral malleolus, but in all other fractures non-weight-bearing will be the norm and all movements absent or greatly reduced.

Figure 9.9 Undisplaced distal fibular fracture (I). The two standard views are normally adequate to demonstrate fractures about the ankle joint, but the fracture will not necessarily appear on both views. In this typical example of a fracture due to an inversion injury, the AP view (left) is unremarkable, and the lateral view (right) shows an oblique fracture of the fibula, which is superimposed over the distal tibia and talus. Check the AP view again: the joint spaces around the talus with the tibia and fibula are even and of expected width, indicating that this is a stable fracture.

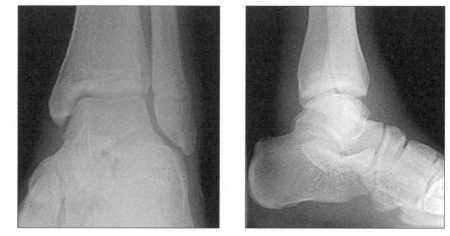

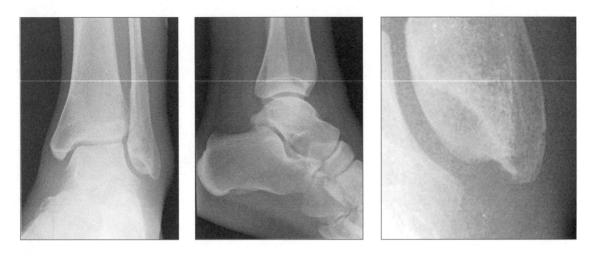

Figure 9.10 (detail view right): Undisplaced distal fibular fracture (II). This injury was again caused by the inversion of the foot and has resulted in an undisplaced fracture of the very tip of the distal fibula. This time it is only visible on the AP view (left) and demonstrates the need for a very careful survey of the bone cortex of all the component bones using appropriate magnification. It cannot be reliably seen on the lateral view (centre).

Treatment

Avulsion fractures are essentially a severe sprain and can be treated with a support bandage, analgesia and gentle exercises. However, if the patient is in severe pain, immobilization in a plaster cast may be required. Oblique/spiral fractures are unstable and are treated in a below-knee non-weight-bearing plaster cast. Displaced fractures (> 1 cm) should be referred, as these may need internal fixation (Dandy and Edwards, 2003).

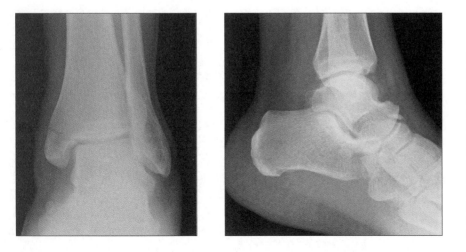

Figure 9.11 Medial malleolar fracture. An intra-articular fracture is clearly seen passing across the medial malleolus and communicating with the tibio-talar joint. It is not seen on the lateral view; but look at the navicular: is this a fracture or an accessory ossification centre?

Figure 9.12 Distal tibial fracture. This patient presented to the X-ray department from his GP after slipping down three steps. He had fractured the postero-medial aspect of his tibia, and the fracture line is seen extending into the joint. On the lateral view (right), the degree of displacement and length of fracture is clearly seen. This patient had been able to carry on with many normal activities, including yoga, for three weeks after injuring himself.

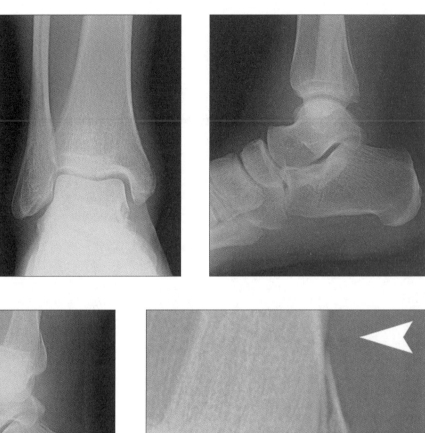

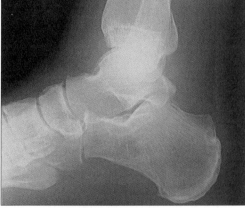

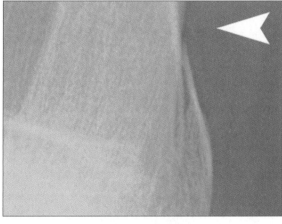

Figure 9.13 Posterior malleolar fracture. This injury was caused by stumbling awkwardly down a step. Abnormalities are seen on both views. The AP view shows an unequal joint space around the talus indicating ligamentous disruption and therefore instability, whereas a break in the cortex of the posterior margin of the distal tibia is seen on the lateral view – white arrowhead on detail view (Figure 9.14 below, bottom left). Because of the superimposition of the tibia and fibula on the lateral projection, this type of fracture is occasionally missed. In fact, positioning in this example is not perfect: the ankle is slightly over-rotated projecting the fibula too far posteriorly and obscuring the individual cortices. The AP view is also abnormal: at the tip of the distal fibula is what appears to be a small avulsion fracture.

Treatment

Most fractures involving the distal tibia and/or medial malleolus are unstable and should be referred for internal fixation. Undisplaced medial malleolus fractures can be treated in a below-knee non-weight-bearing plaster cast.

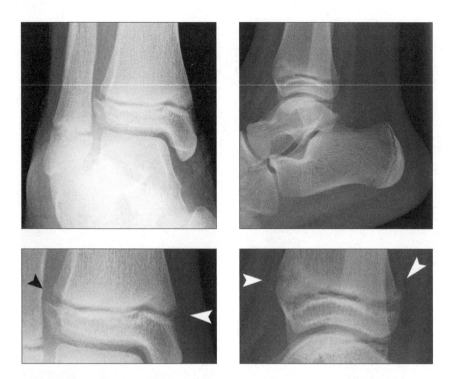

Figure 9.14 Salter and Harris type I fracture, distal tibia (and two detail views below). This would be an extremely easy fracture to miss. This young boy hurt himself while playing football. The epiphysis is very slightly out of normal alignment with the metaphysis; there is a step that is most clearly seen at the posterior aspect of the tibia on the lateral view – see white arrowheads on detail views below. If in doubt, get an experienced opinion of your films. There are many examples of 'steps' in juvenile bones that are as a result of normal development. On the detail AP view (below right), there is a little fragmentation seen at the lateral aspect of the growth plate (black arrowhead), which would, strictly speaking, require that this is reclassified as a Salter and Harris type II fracture, although it is rather an academic point with so tiny a fragment.

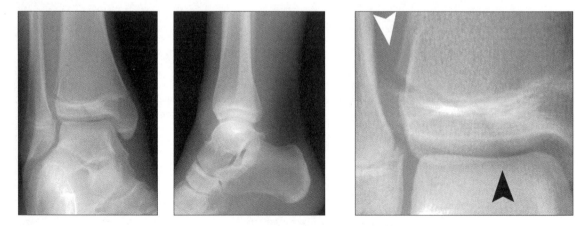

Figure 9.15 (detail view below): This is a tricky fracture to spot and would probably rely on clinical findings and a follow-up X-ray to confirm. There is a fracture through the centre of the distal tibial epiphysis – black arrowhead on detail view (below) – and this has allowed the lateral aspect of the epiphysis to displace slightly – white arrowhead (below). This is classified as a Salter and Harris type III fracture. Note the joint effusion on the lateral view (right).

Comminuted fractures

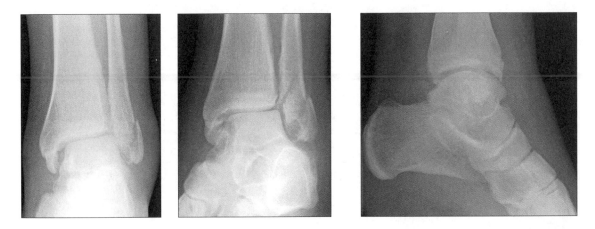

Figure 9.16 Bimalleolar fracture. There is a fracture of the medial malleolus and a spiral fracture of the lateral malleolus. A mortice view has been done (centre) that demonstrates the joint space around the talus well and would indicate any talar shift or syndesmotic disruption. This is an unstable fracture requiring referral and surgical intervention.

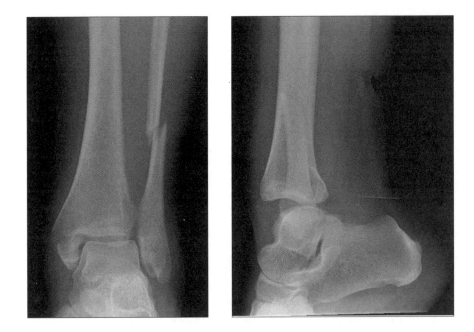

Figure 9.17 Comminuted ankle fracture. There are several components to this injury, which was due to an RTA. Most obvious is the oblique fracture of the fibular shaft with some displacement of the fragments. There is also a fracture across the medial malleolus. Note also that on the AP view (left) the tip of the medial malleolus remains closely applied to the talus, indicating that the ligaments in this region are intact. However, the gap between the distal tibia and fibula is abnormally widened indicating disruption of the interosseous ligament of the syndesmosis. On the lateral view (right), the distal fibula is normally superimposed over the talus, whereas the tibia is subluxed anteriorly. This is an unstable ankle and requires referral for surgical intervention.

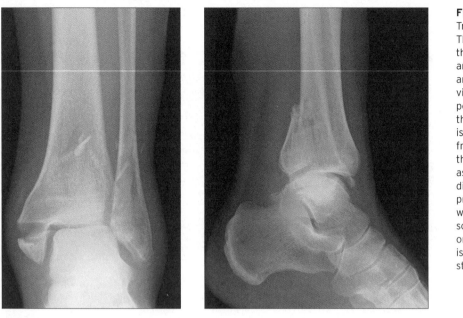

Figure 9.18
Trimalleolar fracture. There is a fracture through the lateral and medial malleoli and, on the lateral view (right), the posterior aspect of the distal tibia. This is an unstable fracture that could therefore be associated with a dislocation on first presentation. Fixing with plates and screws by an orthopaedic surgeon is required to restore stability.

Tibial and fibular midshaft fractures

Isolated fractures to the tibia or fibula can occur, but mainly as a result of direct trauma. Twisting injuries can lead to isolated fractures of the fibula. However, fracture to the proximal fibula is associated with a distal tibial fracture (the so-called 'Maisonneuve' fracture, although strictly speaking this includes a disruption of the distal tibio-fibular syndesmosis) and, consequently, the ankle, the tibial and fibular shafts and the knee must be examined. Stress fractures can occur in long-distance runners (affecting the tibia and fibula) or male ballet dancers (tibia) (Dandy and Edwards, 2003). Much more common are fractures both to the tibia and fibula, especially through RTAs and twisting-sports injuries (e.g. snow boarding).

As the tibia lies subcutaneously, it is at risk of an open fracture and wound care is extremely important to prevent osteomyolitis. Stem any bleeding. Note any obvious deformity, swelling or bruising. Ensure the fibular head, tibial plateau and all the bones in the ankle are palpated in addition to the shafts of the tibia and fibula. Ensure any tenderness away from the obvious injury site is noted on the X-ray request form – otherwise the whole limb and joint above/below may not be included on the radiograph. Check the neurovascular status of the foot as these injuries run a high risk of nerve and/or vascular damage. The patient is unlikely to weight-bear except in fibular head fractures and stress fractures. Evaluate all ankle movements.

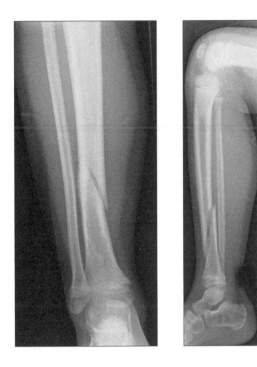

Figure 9.19 Spiral fracture to the tibial shaft. This young boy was injured while playing football and the result is a spiral fracture of the tibial shaft. Always check the entire length of the tibial and fibular shafts; a neck-of-fibular fracture would not be a surprising finding.

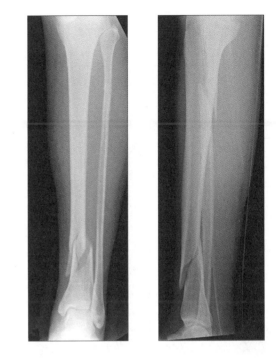

Figure 9.20 There is a spiral fracture of the distal tibia with some degree of rotation. However, there is also a fracture of the proximal fibula. In the event of distal tibial injuries, a fracture of the proximal third of the fibula should be suspected due to the principle of the 'ring of bone' or 'contre-coup' injury. Where there is a fracture in a ring of bone such as the combined tibia and fibula or the mandible, one fracture occurring can often mean that a second fracture is present as the bone ring tends to break in two places. This is often termed a Maisonneuve fracture – although this also involves a disruption of the distal tibio-fibular syndesmosis.

Treatment

Undisplaced, isolated shaft/head fractures of the fibula are treated conservatively if the ankle movements are not too painful. Otherwise, plaster-cast immobilization is indicated. Stress fractures are always immobilized. Tibial shaft fractures are treated the same whether or not the fibula is injured. Any wounds are cleaned and covered and the fracture is usually always fixed either internally or externally. Any displaced fractures are reduced prior to immobilization.

Undisplaced, stable fractures are treated in a plaster cast and regularly followed up.

Toddler fractures

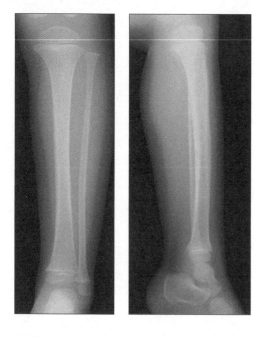

Figure 9.21 Toddler fracture. There is a faint lucent line seen running obliquely across the distal tibia on both views in this examination. This is a classic injury occurring to young children learning to walk: they may overbalance or wobble and fall, the body twists while the foot remains firmly on the ground. The twisting force produces the fracture. These can sometimes be very difficult to pick out (see Figure 9.22, below).

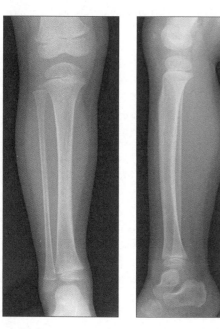

Figure 9.22 (detail view below): Another toddler fracture with the same mechanism of injury as in the previous example. This time the fracture is almost invisible on the lateral view (right) and completely undetectable on the AP view (left). In this case, the child was completely refusing to walk. A very careful close look at the film reveals the faint fracture line that is not even seen to cross the bone cortex; however, it is definitely a fracture (see detail view), and a follow-up film will undoubtedly reveal periosteal reaction and callus formation as healing and repair take place.

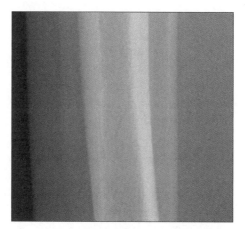

Calcaneal fractures

Calcaneal fractures are usually sustained as a result of landing on the heel from a height but can occur from a twisting injury (Dandy and Edwards, 2003). The calcaneus is made up of cancellous bone that crushes upon impact (Dandy and Edwards, 2003). If the forces involved are of a great enough magnitude, the energy is transferred upwards and patients should always have their knees, hips and lumbar region examined routinely (McRae, 1999). The Achilles tendon inserts into the posterior aspect of the calcaneus, and a ruptured Achilles tendon may avulse bone off the calcaneus. A ruptured Achilles tendon is essentially a clinical diagnosis and calcaneus X-rays are not routinely obtained.

Look

Often the other calcaneus is also fractured, and it is essential to examine both limbs. The heel may appear wider, shorter, flatter and may have a lateral tilt into a valgus. Swelling is usually present and may be extensive. Bruising takes a day or so to appear and spreads to the sole of the foot in a horseshoe pattern. If a complete Achilles tendon rupture is suspected, there is a loss of the normal contour of the tendon.

Feel

There will be severe tenderness on palpation and squeezing of the heel from the sides. A palpable gap may be felt over the Achilles tendon if ruptured, but is not always present.

Move

The patient is usually non-weight-bearing. Fractures to the calcaneus can disrupt the subtalar joint, which is where inversion/eversion takes place. Consequently, these movements are restricted and painful. If a ruptured Achilles tendon is suspected, the patient will be unable to weight-bear on the front of the foot, but may still be able to plantar-flex due to the actions of the flexor hallucis longus and the toe flexors. This will be weaker and may be painful. The Simmonds test must be undertaken when a ruptured Achilles tendon is suspected. The patient kneels on a chair (or lies flat on a couch) with both ankles over the end of the chair/couch. The calf muscle is squeezed and the plantar-flexion of the foot noted. The test is positive (i.e. the Achilles tendon is assumed to be ruptured) if the plantar-flexion is absent or reduced. Always compare with the other leg.

Calcaneal radiographs can be difficult to interpret, and it is important to indicate on the X-ray request form that a calcaneal fracture is suspected to ensure an axial view is obtained. This view is centred on the base of the heel with the foot dorsi-flexed as much as the patient can bear and with the X-ray beam angled up towards the head.

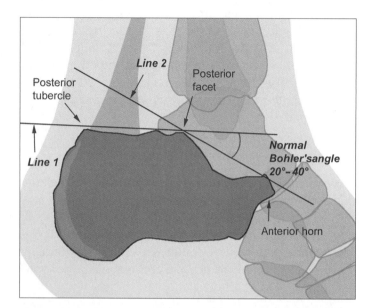

Figure 9.23 Bohler's angle. The calcaneus is irregularly shaped. However, there is a useful tool that can assist in detecting subtle fractures. Two lines can be drawn on the lateral view of the calcaneus. Line one joins the highest point of the posterior tuberosity to the apex of the posterior facet and line two joins the apex of the posterior facet to the tip of the anterior horn, as shown in the diagram. The angle is variable but the normal range is 20°–40°. An angle of less than 20° is suggestive of fracture through the posterior facet, and the radiographs should be scrutinized for evidence of fracture.

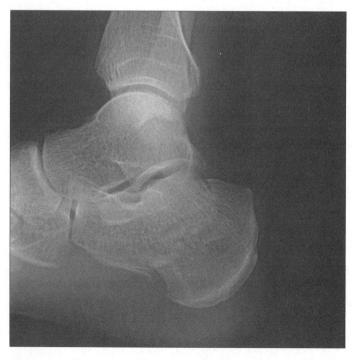

Figure 9.24 Calcaneal fracture. There is a fracture through the posterior aspect of the calcaneus that intersects with the posterior facet superiorly. The posterior fragment has shifted upward and this gives a flatter than normal Bohler's angle. The overlap of the fracture fragments also shows as increased density along the fracture line.

Figure 9.25 Gross calcaneal fracture seen on lateral (left) and axial view (right). This injury occurred after this young man jumped from a height of about 20 feet and landed on his feet. Both calcanei suffered similar crush fractures. It is not uncommon in accidents involving this much energy for the spine to be injured – due consideration should therefore be given to requesting lumbar or thoracic spine X-rays as appropriate.

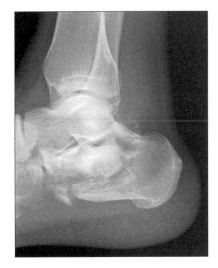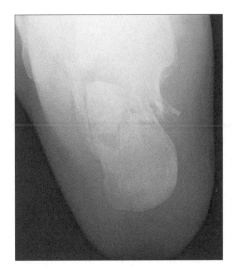

Figure 9.26 Calcaneal anterior horn fracture. This is an easy fracture to miss due to other overlying structures. There is a fracture of the anterior horn or process in the region of the articulation with the navicular and cuboid. Always trace around the entire cortex of each bone looking for a step deformity.

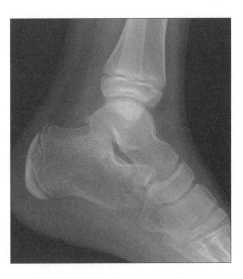

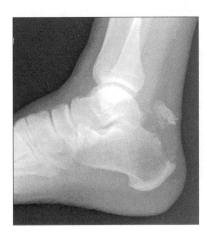

Figure 9.27 Avulsion fracture of the Achilles insertion. The posterior tuberosity of the calcaneus has been avulsed, although part of the insertion of the Achilles tendon does appear to be intact.

Treatment

All calcaneal fractures should be discussed with the orthopaedic surgeons as the patient may need admission for elevation. A ruptured Achilles tendon is either treated in a non-weight-bearing plaster cast (with foot in acquaneus position) or surgically repaired.

Talar injuries

The talus has an important role in three joints: ankle, subtalar and talo-navicular. Given that up to half of all talar neck fractures result in avascular necrosis, injuries to this bone can have severe consequences for the future function of both the ankle and the foot (McRae, 1999). The mechanism of injury is usually through forced dorsi-flexion (e.g. in RTA), a fall from a height or twisting injuries (Dandy and Edwards, 2003; McRae, 1999). There is often diffuse swelling, and deformity may be present depending on the severity of the injury. Observe the skin integrity as this may necroze if under pressure. Pain will be severe and can be difficult to isolate from surrounding bones. Check distal neurovascular function. The patient will be non-weight-bearing and all movements are restricted and painful.

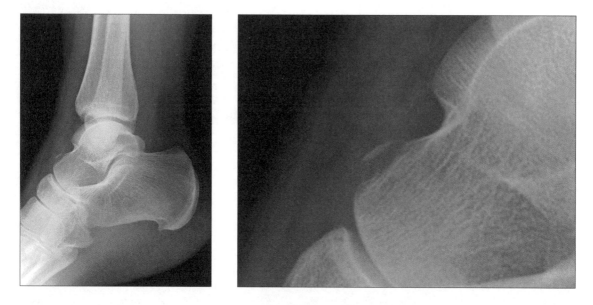

Figure 9.28 Dorsal talar fracture. There is a flake fragment of bone seen on the lateral view from the tip of the talus anteriorly.

Figure 9.29
Another talar flake fracture – white arrow on detail view (right). This time there is also a large joint effusion within the joint capsule (outlined by white arrowheads).

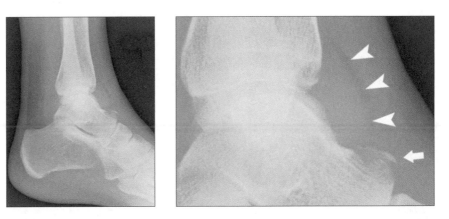

Figure 9.30 Medial talar fracture. A small fragment of bone is seen to have detached from the medial aspect of the talus just below the tip of the medial malleolus on the AP view (left). It is undisplaced and is not seen on the lateral view.

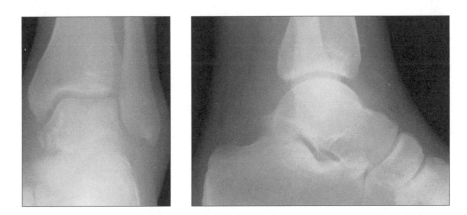

Figure 9.31 Talar fracture dislocation. This is a serious injury with complete fracture of the talus. The anterior fragment has maintained articulation with the navicular, but the posterior part has displaced backward and rotated. Referral and surgical intervention are the only course of action. Note the completely disrupted joint space on the AP view (left).

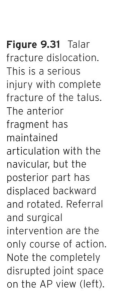
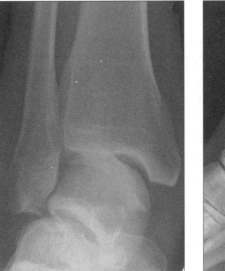
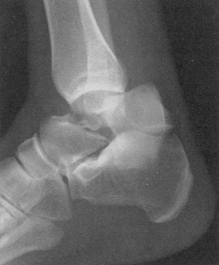

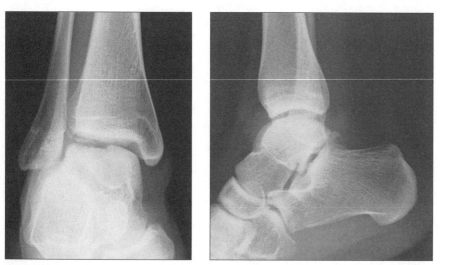

Figure 9.32 Impacted tibial and talar fracture. The fractures are well seen on the AP view (left). Scrutiny of the joint space reveals crush-type disruption to the normally smooth articular surface of both talus and distal tibia caused by falling from a height onto the foot. The calcaneus (lateral view, right) is intact, but note the joint effusion.

Treatment

All talar fractures (apart from the dorsal flake fractures) are serious and should be referred to the orthopaedic surgeons, as several complications can occur:

- skin necrosis if talus is displaced – early reduction is essential
- non-union
- avascular necrosis if the fracture is through the neck of the talus
- osteoarthritis of subtalar and talo-navicular joints
- osteochondral fragments
- open fractures leading to sepsis

Figure 9.33 Both of these examples show fractures that are detectable on the lateral ankle views, but they are normally better demonstrated on foot views. The left-hand view shows an undisplaced fracture at the base of the fifth metatarsal, and the right-hand view shows a fractured navicular. Always include these regions in your scan of ankle views. See Chapter 10 for details of treatments.

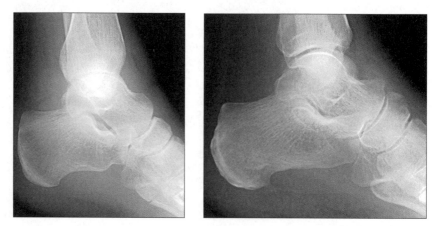

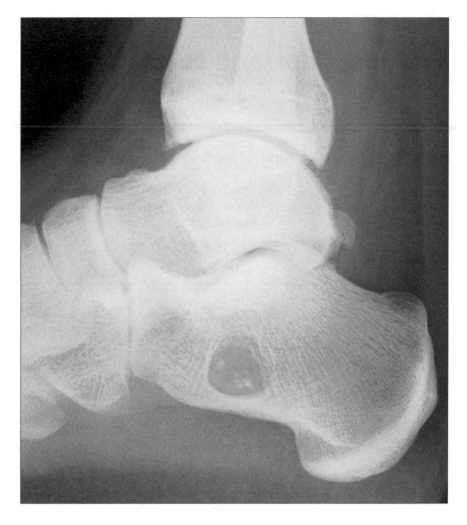

Figure 9.34 Pseudocyst. This is an occasional finding in images of the calcaneus. A cystic appearance often occurs at this junction of three trabecular patterns and is an absence of the normal trabecular bone in this region. Although this is not a sinister finding in this case, all lesions should be checked by a radiologist in case further investigation is required.

Chapter 10

The fore-foot and toes

Review of core anatomy

In addition to supporting body weight, the foot also acts as a shock absorber and is essential for walking, running and maintaining balance. The foot consists of 28 bones grouped together in three parts:

- the hind-foot: talus and calcaneus (discussed in previous chapter)
- the mid-foot: cuboid, navicular and the three cuneiforms
- the fore-foot: metatarsals and phalanges

The foot consists of several, mainly small, joints held tightly together by ligaments, allowing little movements between them. The most important joints are (Dean and Pegington, 1996):

- subtalar joint (discussed in previous chapter)
- talo-calcaneal joint (discussed in previous chapter)
- talo-navicular joint
- calcaneo-cuboid joint
- tarso-metatarsal joint

The talo-navicular joint is anatomically a ball-and-socket joint, although there is not the usual amount of movement normally associated with this type of joint (Dean and Pegington, 1996). Between the bones lies the spring ligament, which helps form the medial longitudinal arch of the foot (Dean and Pegington, 1996). The calcaneus and the cuboid articulate in a synovial joint, strengthened by several ligaments, especially the long plantar ligament, which also plays an important role in forming and maintaining the arches of the foot (Dean and Pegington, 1996; Moore, 1992). The tarso-metatarsal joint separates the mid-foot from the fore-foot and is formed by the articulation of the metatarsals with the cuboid and the cuneiforms in a synovial-type joint, which allows some gliding movement. This joint is sometimes referred to as 'Lisfranc' joint.

The navicular is a flat boat-shaped bone, lying between the head of the talus and the three cuneiforms. There is also some articulation with the cuboid. The cuboid is a wedge-shaped bone and is the most laterally lying of the mid-foot bones. It articulates posteriorly with the calcaneus, anteriorly with the fourth and fifth metatarsals and medially with the lateral cuneiform and navicular. The three cuneiforms are described as medial (the largest), intermediate (smallest) and lateral.

The metatarsals are numbered 1 to 5, with the metatarsal of the hallux being number 1. They are long bones, and thus have a base (proximally), which articulate with the cuneiforms and cuboids, and a shaft and a head (distally), which articulates with the phalanges at the metatarso-phalangeal joints. Around the head of the first metatarsal lie the lateral and medial sesamoid bones, which aid the first metatarsal head during part of walking. The second metatarsal sits slightly higher dorsally and is more vulnerable to crush injuries. The base of the fifth metatarsal has a large tuberosity providing attachment to the peroneous brevis tendon. Rupture of the peroneous brevis tendon causes a commonly encountered avulsion fracture.

The foot bones are arranged to form the longitudinal (composed of the calcaneus, talus, navicular, cuneiforms and metatarsals) and the transverse (runs from side to side and is composed of the cuboid, three cuneiforms and the base of the metatarsals) arches necessary to enable the foot to adapt to changes in the surface or weight. When walking, the weight of the body is transferred from the tibia to the talus, then to the calcaneus and finally to the heads of the metatarsals. The talus is often described as the 'key stone' as it is the first foot bone to receive the weight of the body (Moore, 1992; Dean and Pegington, 1996).

The foot receives its blood supply from the anterior and posterior tibial artery (divisions of the popliteal artery), with further subdivision into several branches, some of which joins on the dorsum of the foot to form an arch. The nerve supply to the lower leg is complex but has five terminal branches supplying the ankle and foot. Consequently, the whole of the foot must be thoroughly assessed to ensure the integrity of all the branches.

Clinical examination

The foot is vulnerable to crush injuries either from being trapped (e.g. Under a foot-pedal in RTAs), heavy objects being dropped onto it or from being run over by various vehicles. Crush injuries can be severe even in the absence of fractures, as compartment syndrome can occur in the small muscles (Wardrope and English, 1998). Stress fractures are not uncommon and usually occur when a person starts new, strenuous activities. It is often described as a 'march' fracture as it was commonly seen in new soldiers (Dean and Pegington, 1996).

Look

Swelling can be excessive and can lead to compartment syndrome. It is useful to obtain the approximate weight of the object in crush injuries. The mid-foot bones are well splinted and held tightly together by several ligaments, and deformities may not be immediately obvious to see. Observe toe nails for subungual haematomas, and drain if necessary.

Feel

Palpate all bones in the foot and toes for tenderness, including the joint above. Pay particular attention to the navicular and the base of the fifth metatarsal, as these bones commonly fracture. Ensure neurovascular assessment is undertaken by evaluating sensation, pulses and capillary refill in the foot.

Move

Most movements of the foot take place at the subtalar joint (see Chapter 9 for details of injuries to the ankle). With the foot plantar-flexed, inversion (30°) and eversion (10°) can take place. At the metatarso-phalangeal joints, extension (dorsi-flexion) of approximately 60° and flexion (plantar-flexion) of 40° take places.

Ottawa ankle rules

The Ottawa ankle rules (Steill et al., 1995) are based upon decision-making criteria regarding the need for an X-ray and have been extensively studied and validated. The rules seek to determine if an X-ray

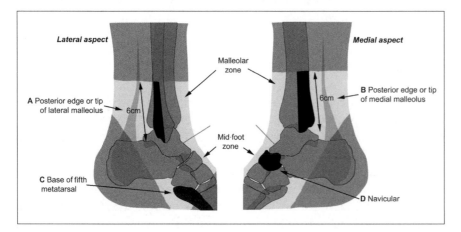

Figure 10.1 Ottawa ankle rules (Steill et al., 1995). (Reproduced with kind permission, BMJ Publishing Group)

is indicated and, if so, whether an ankle or a foot X-ray is to be requested, as rarely both are needed. This rule should be consulted in any foot injuries.

An X-ray series of the foot is required only if there is any pain in the mid-foot zone and any of these findings:

bone tenderness at C
bone tenderness at D
inability to bear weight both immediately and when examined

Standard projections

DP
DP oblique

Additional projections

lateral foot (for foreign-body localization or occasionally an orthopaedic request)

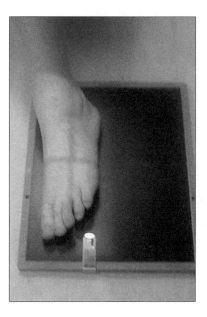

Figure 10.2 X-ray positioning of the DP oblique view of the foot.

X-ray positioning

Positioning of the foot is straightforward: the patient sits on the X-ray table with the knee flexed and the plantar surface of the foot flat on the cassette. The view should include from the entire foot and tarsal bones; however, the talus and calcaneus are not usefully demonstrated on the DP view. For the DP oblique view, the lateral aspect of the foot is raised and the knee rotated past the midline such that the lower leg is at an angle of about 45° to the table. The DP oblique view does demonstrate the talus and calcaneus a little better, but these bones are better visualized with ankle and/or calcaneal views. The foot is a wedge-shaped structure with a much greater density of tissue towards the ankle and less towards the toes. This results in a radiograph where the toes may be over-penetrated, whereas the tarsal bones can be under-penetrated by the X-ray beam, and consequently produce an image that fails to demonstrate all the anatomy adequately. Wedge filters are available that are placed on the X-ray cassette and can even out this differential in density and improve the quality of the image.

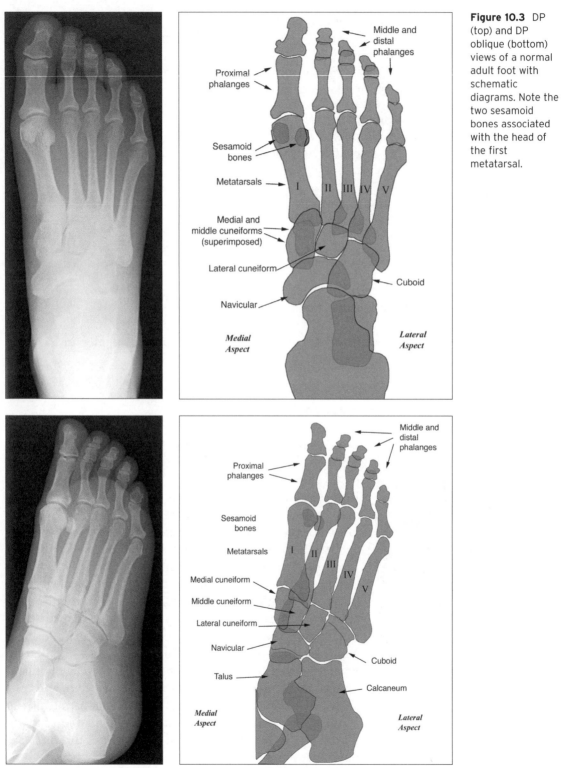

Figure 10.3 DP (top) and DP oblique (bottom) views of a normal adult foot with schematic diagrams. Note the two sesamoid bones associated with the head of the first metatarsal.

Radiographic interpretation

Interpretation of foot radiographs can be confusing, and it is possible to miss fractures as the views are complex with many overlying structures. As always, try and develop a systematic and structured scan of the images. From personal experience, the foot is probably the region where there is most likely to be more than one fracture; so, if an abnormality is detected, always continue with your search until you have examined all of the anatomy.

Trace around the cortex of each bone individually; the distal phalanges of the little toes are often fused and this is a normal variant. In the juvenile foot, the shape of the physis at the base of the first metatarsal and the proximal phalanx of the great toe is irregular and can be mistaken for a fracture. There are prominent sesamoid bones associated with the metatarso-phalangeal joint of the great toe and these are occasionally bipartite (i.e. ossify from two separate centres of ossification), although a sesamoid bone can also fracture in its own right. Pay particular attention to the metatarsal head and neck; these are susceptible to fracture, e.g. from a stubbing injury, but can be very hard to detect. The metatarsals articulate at their bases with each other and with the tarsals; excessive gaps between the bases of the metatarsals can indicate dislocation and/or fracture of the associated tarsal.

The hind-foot is confusing to the novice due to the overlapping of structures; however, look carefully at both views and identify all the anatomy – the tarsals can look very different in the two views. Note that the medial border of the second metatarsal aligns with the articulation between the medial and middle cuneiforms on the DP view; on the DP oblique view, the lateral border of the second metatarsal aligns with the articulation between the middle and lateral cuneiforms. This is fine in theory, but in practice it is difficult to remember this alignment. However, a cuneiform fracture can result in the disruption of the normal appearance of the base of the metatarsals (see Figure 10.11). If a rule is difficult to remember, don't try and remember it – you can always look it up when the need arises.

There are many extra bones (accessory ossicles) in the foot that can be seen as normal variants, some are named – see Keats (1996). Accessory ossicles are well rounded and have a defined bony cortex that distinguishes them from fractures from the adjacent bone. In the juvenile bone, the tuberosity of the base of the fifth metatarsal forms as a separate *apophysis* (as distinct from an *epiphysis*) but it is distinguished from a fracture of the metatarsal as it aligns with the long axis of the bone; a fracture of the base of the fifth metatarsal is *across* the long axis of the bone.

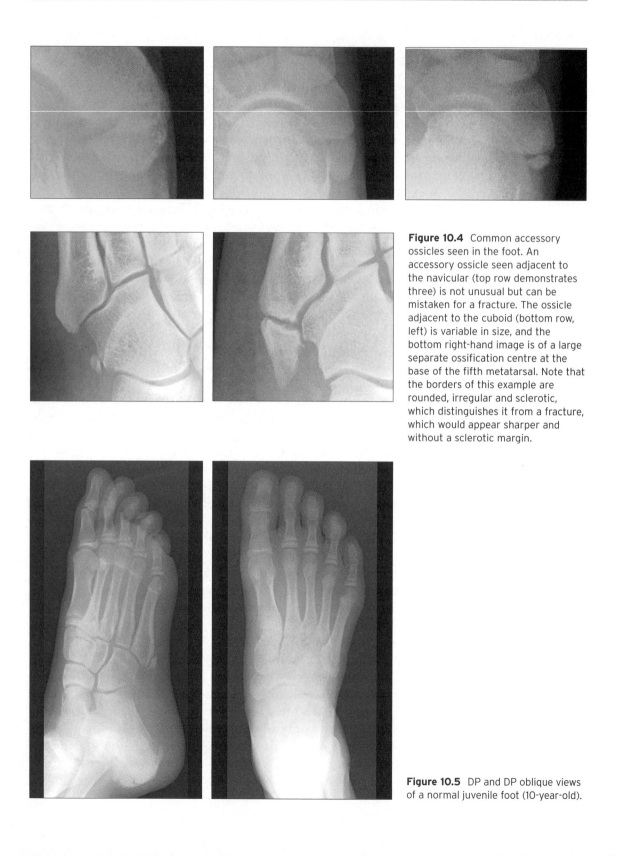

Figure 10.4 Common accessory ossicles seen in the foot. An accessory ossicle seen adjacent to the navicular (top row demonstrates three) is not unusual but can be mistaken for a fracture. The ossicle adjacent to the cuboid (bottom row, left) is variable in size, and the bottom right-hand image is of a large separate ossification centre at the base of the fifth metatarsal. Note that the borders of this example are rounded, irregular and sclerotic, which distinguishes it from a fracture, which would appear sharper and without a sclerotic margin.

Figure 10.5 DP and DP oblique views of a normal juvenile foot (10-year-old).

In the juvenile foot, there is a profusion of epiphyses making the radiographs more complex to examine (Figure 10.5). Note in this example there is a very prominent apophysis at the base of the fifth metatarsal; however, the direction is in line with the long axis of the bone and is irregular and somewhat fragmented. These findings differentiate this from a fracture. The metatarsal epiphysis of the big toe is at the base, whereas in the second to fifth toes the epiphyses are at the heads of the metatarsals. This is a similar arrangement to that seen in the metacarpals of the hand. The epiphyses at the base of the toes are broad and flat and can appear unusually dense – i.e. bright white – but this is only due to the high concentration of cortical bone.

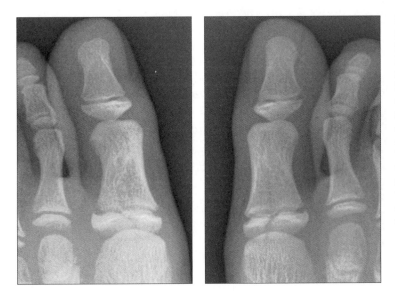

Figure 10.6 Bipartite epiphysis at the base of the proximal phalanx of the great toes. This 11-year-old boy had his left foot X-rayed following a stubbing injury. The appearance was initially taken for a fracture; a comparison view of the other foot shows an almost identical appearance, thus discounting this as a fracture. The epiphysis has formed from two separate ossification centres resulting in a cleft in the middle, which mimics a fracture. Note the absence of soft-tissue swelling and an accurate alignment of the epiphyseal margins.

Fractures to the mid-foot (tarsal fractures)

The navicular commonly sustains an avulsion fracture of its tuberosity; otherwise the mid-foot bones are not easily fractured (except following crush injuries) as they are held tightly together by complex joints, ligaments and muscles.

A rare but easily missed injury is a dislocation or a fracture/dislocation of the mid-tarsal joint, formed by the talus and calcaneus posteriorly and the navicular and cuboid anteriorly. In this injury, the talus and calcaneus lose their normal articulation with the navicular and cuboid bones. The mechanism of injury can be a relatively minor twisting movement, although it can also occur following a fall from a height or an RTA. This injury should not be mistaken for the tarso-metatarsal dislocation (with or without a fracture), known as the 'Lisfranc' injury (see Figure 10.13). In a Lisfranc injury, the metatarsals dislocate away (usually laterally) from their normal articulation with the mid-tarsal bones, putting the foot at risk of vascular compromise, as the foot's arterial supply crosses the tarso-metatarsal joint. This injury can be quite subtle and easily missed, especially if there is no accompanying fracture. Check the normal alignment of the metatarsals with the cuneiforms and have a higher index of suspicion of a dislocation (or subluxation) if bony fragments have detached from the base of the metatarsals. The mechanism of injury for a Lisfranc dislocation is similar to the dislocation of the mid-tarsal joint, and includes twisting movements, falls onto the foot while dorsi-flexed, RTAs (especially with foot trapped in dorsi-flexion under a foot pedal) and crush injuries.

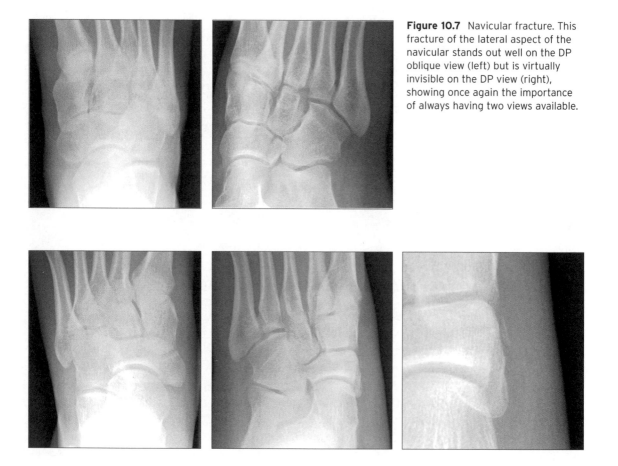

Figure 10.7 Navicular fracture. This fracture of the lateral aspect of the navicular stands out well on the DP oblique view (left) but is virtually invisible on the DP view (right), showing once again the importance of always having two views available.

Figure 10.8 Flake fracture of the medial aspect of the navicular. Again, this fracture is only seen on the DP oblique view.

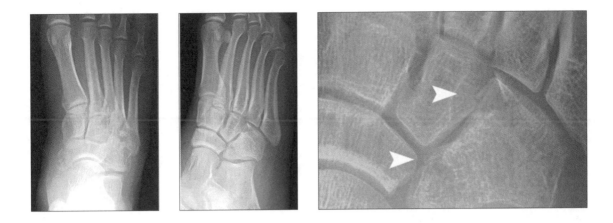

Figure 10.9 Fracture of the medial aspect of the navicular and comminuted fracture of the cuboid – white arrowheads, detail view (bottom). This injury occurred as a result of a trip with a stumbling, twisting action. It would be easy to miss the cuboid element of the injury after successfully spotting the navicular fracture. However, this is a serious injury requiring orthopaedic referral; secondary osteoarthritis is a likely outcome, but this patient had six months away from work while the fractures healed sufficiently to weight-bear for long periods.

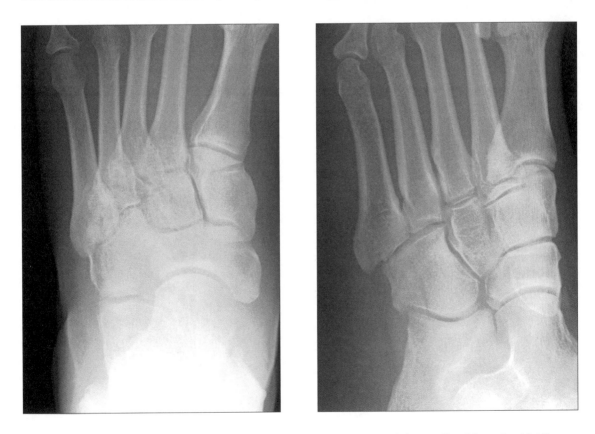

Figure 10.10 Cuboid fracture. This undisplaced fracture of the cuboid is more obvious on the oblique view (right), which demonstrates a joint space all around the cuboid allowing for a good scrutiny of the bony cortex.

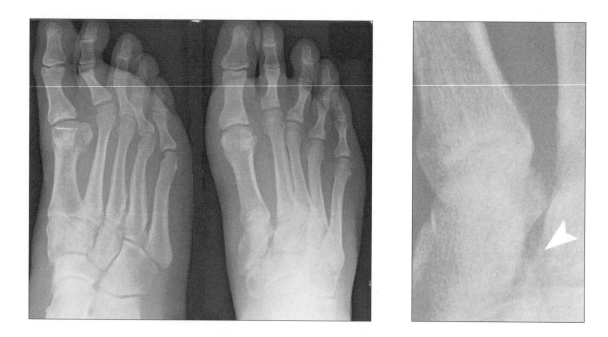

Figure 10.11 (detail view right): This fracture is of the medial cuneiform — see white arrowhead on the detail view. Attention should be drawn to this region by the abnormally wide gap between the first and second metatarsals, particularly on the DP view. When this is evident, you must look very carefully at all the tarsal bones to identify the cause. In fact, these films were taken three weeks post-injury (a fall), when presumably partial weight-bearing had increased the fracture separation and widened the gap between the metatarsals.

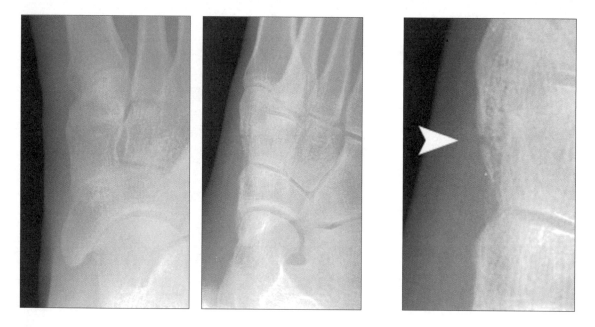

Figure 10.12 Another medial cuneiform fracture. This time there is a break in the medial cortical margin, which, once again, is only visible on the DP oblique detail view — arrowhead.

Figure 10.13 Lisfranc fracture dislocation at the junction of the mid-foot and fore-foot. This is a serious unstable injury requiring orthopaedic referral. Note the widened gap between the first and second metatarsals and the loss of articulation between the base of the fifth metatarsal and the cuboid; the second to fourth metatarsals have slipped laterally compromising the stability of the entire foot.

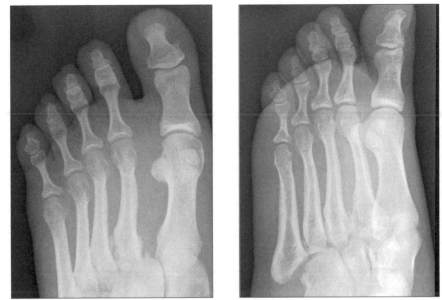

Treatment

Isolated fractures to the mid-foot bones are treated conservatively in a non-weight-bearing plaster cast. The patient must be instructed to adequately elevate the limb to help reduce swelling. Avulsion fractures to the navicular are treated in a supportive bandage with advice to keep the foot elevated and ice therapy to help reduce swelling.

A comfortable and supportive shoe/boot is the best 'splint' that can be used. If the patient is in severe pain, a short period of plaster immobilization may be used. Dislocations must be reduced as soon as possible to prevent vascular compromise, and immediate referral to orthopaedics is indicated.

Metatarsal fractures

The most common metatarsal fracture is an avulsion fracture to the base of the fifth metatarsal, where the peroneous brevis tendon avulses off its bony attachment during forced inversion. This injury is frequently confused with the so-called Jones' fracture (fracture to the fifth metatarsal distal to the tuberosity), but it is important to distinguish the two, as not only is the mechanism of injury different but so is also the treatment. A Jones' fracture is not caused by an inversion injury but is usually seen in athletic 15- to 21-year-olds. A Jones' fracture is now often (wrongly) used to describe any fifth-metatarsal fractures that are not to the base/tuberosity, but a true Jones' fracture, as described by Sir Robert Jones, an orthopaedic surgeon, in 1903 who described a fracture his foot sustained while dancing, is a fracture at the junction of the proximal metaphysis and diaphysis.

Fractures to the shaft and neck of the metatarsals tend to occur following crush injuries, but spiral fractures are also seen after forced inversion or eversion of the foot. Beware of the stress (also known as march or fatigue) fracture. Usually, it is the second metatarsal neck that is involved and the fracture is usually diagnosed by callus formation. The patient will generally complain of pain for a few weeks and localized tenderness, but has no clear history of trauma. Instead, a recent period of new or increased strenuous activities is identified.

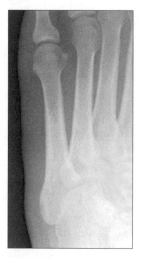
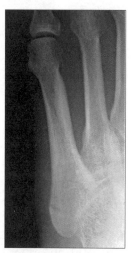
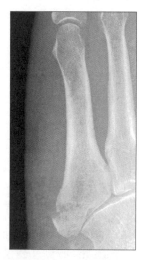

Figure 10.14 Three examples of fractures of the base of the fifth metatarsal increasing left to right in degree of displacement. This fracture is one of the most commonly seen in the foot and is normally the result of an inversion injury. The strong peroneous brevis tendon attaches to the base of the fifth metatarsal and during the inversion of the foot pulls at the bone, which fractures horizontally. The degree of displacement of this depends on the mechanical force applied and the integrity of the bone tissue. If the displacement is severe, surgical intervention is required to ensure fracture union. If in doubt, seek advice.

Figure 10.15 A Jones' fracture. This is a fracture of the proximal shaft of the fifth metatarsal and not the base. The mechanism of injury as well as the site are different. It occurs within the proximal 1.5 cm of the shaft as a result of a laterally directed force with the heel off the ground. It can fail to unite or may re-fracture following initial union. It is therefore an indication for orthopaedic referral.

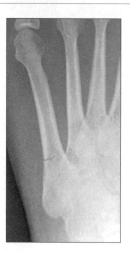
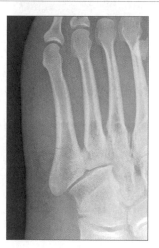

Figure 10.16 Fracture of the base of the third metatarsal. The fracture line is widened and somewhat 'woolly' looking as the film was taken two weeks post-injury (tripping down one step) and this has allowed some bone re-absorption to occur at the fracture site, which has increased the width of the fracture.

Figure 10.17 This fracture at the base of the second metatarsal affects the articulation between the second and third metatarsals. This will cause secondary osteoarthritis to occur post-healing.

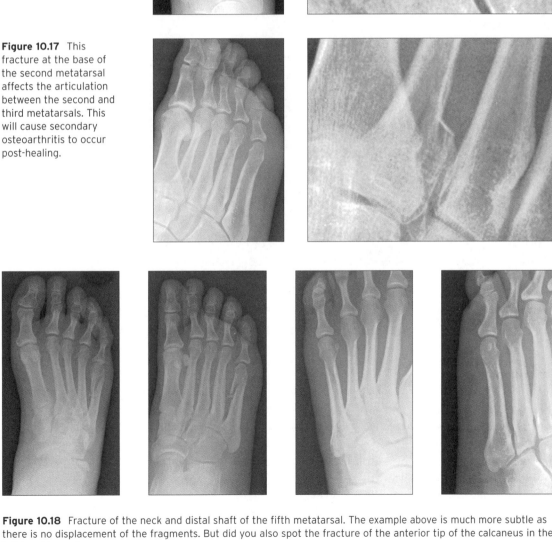

Figure 10.18 Fracture of the neck and distal shaft of the fifth metatarsal. The example above is much more subtle as there is no displacement of the fragments. But did you also spot the fracture of the anterior tip of the calcaneus in the left-hand image?

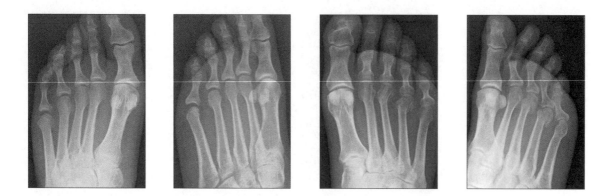

Figure 10.19 (above and below): Fractures of the metatarsal heads are notoriously easy to miss. Those shown below the third and fourth metatarsals are obvious but those shown above are very missable. Check the cortex in this region very carefully for even the tiniest steps or jaggedness.

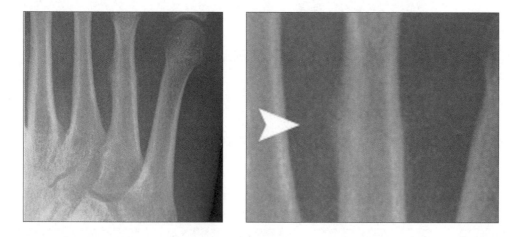

Figure 10.20 The march fracture. This is an absolutely classic fracture where the patient presents many days or even weeks post-injury with chronic pain. The appearance of an indistinct and greyish cortex is actually a representation of the healing process of a fracture that is not itself shown.

Treatment

Avulsion fractures to the base of the fifth metatarsal are treated in a supportive bandage with advice to keep the foot elevated, ice therapy to help reduce swelling and gentle exercise. A comfortable and supportive shoe/boot is the best 'splint' that can be used. If the patient is in severe pain, a short period of plaster immobilization may be used.

Jones' fractures are treated in a non-weight-bearing plaster cast and with orthopaedic follow-up. Occasionally, internal fixation is required. Stress fractures can be treated with rest and reassurance, but occasionally a period of immobilization because of pain can be used.

Most other metatarsal fractures are undisplaced, but even a high degree of displacement is accepted, and single metatarsal fractures are treated either supportively or in a plaster cast if very painful. Multiple metatarsal fractures should be discussed with orthopaedics.

Fractures of the toes

The toes are vulnerable to crush or stubbing injuries and commonly dislocate. X-raying toes 2 to 5 is rarely undertaken as the treatment doesn't alter if the toe is clinically suspected of being fractured. Explain this to the patient and reassure them that the clinically suspected fracture will heal without X-ray. X-ray toes that look obviously deformed. The hallux is essential for normal gait and is always X-rayed.

Subungual haematomas are common and should be drained to relieve pain. Swelling and bruising may be excessive, especially if late presentation and open fractures are common. The patient is usually able to partially weight-bear on the back of the foot.

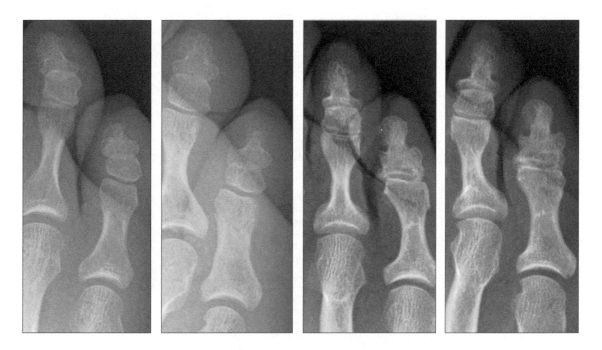

Figure 10.21 Toe fractures are common and most are easy to spot, although occasionally they can be very subtle. However, do not be fooled by its appearance in the third image. This is actually a soft-tissue shadow overlying the proximal phalanx of the little toe, which mimics a fracture. The line can be seen to extend beyond the margins of the bone, and on the oblique view (far right) it is seen in a different position altogether.

Figure 10.22 This transverse fracture of the proximal phalanx of the third toe is obvious on the DP oblique view (left) but is practically invisible on the DP view (right), again reinforcing the need for two views of the region under suspicion.

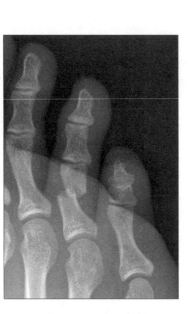

Figure 10.23 This is a comminuted fracture of the distal phalanx of the great toe caused by dropping a heavy weight onto the foot.

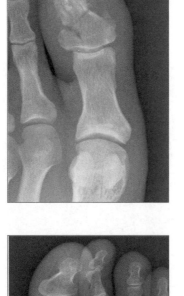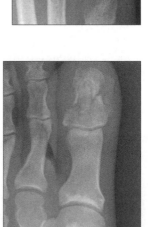

Figure 10.24 The second metatarso-phalangeal joint is clearly dislocated, but there is also a fracture of the neck and distal shaft of the third metatarsal.

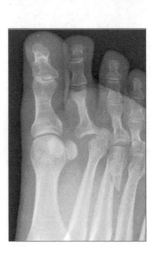

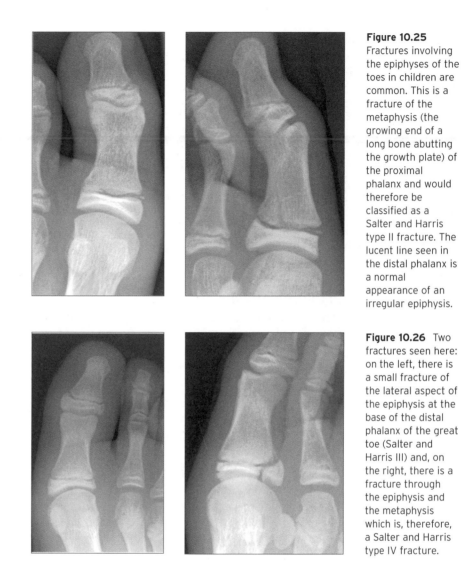

Figure 10.25 Fractures involving the epiphyses of the toes in children are common. This is a fracture of the metaphysis (the growing end of a long bone abutting the growth plate) of the proximal phalanx and would therefore be classified as a Salter and Harris type II fracture. The lucent line seen in the distal phalanx is a normal appearance of an irregular epiphysis.

Figure 10.26 Two fractures seen here: on the left, there is a small fracture of the lateral aspect of the epiphysis at the base of the distal phalanx of the great toe (Salter and Harris III) and, on the right, there is a fracture through the epiphysis and the metaphysis which is, therefore, a Salter and Harris type IV fracture.

Treatment

Pay particular attention to any open fractures and ensure they are thoroughly cleaned and dressed. Prophylactic antibiotics may be required. All injuries to the toes benefit from elevation and ice to reduce swelling.

Clinically fractured toes without any deformity (or gross angulation if X-ray has been obtained) are treated in a neighbour strap and supportive footwear. Gross angulation is reduced, neighbour-strapped and X-rayed again. Dislocations are reduced and X-rayed again post-reduction.

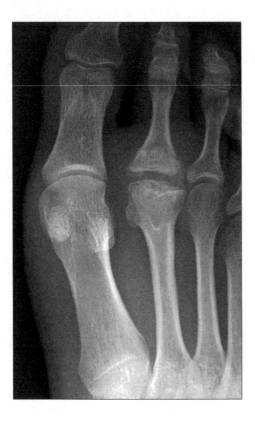

Figure 10.27 To complete the chapter, we have an example of an occasional finding in the metatarso-phalangeal joint of the second toe. This is known as Freiberg's infraction, and the appearances are of a distorted irregular joint with a widening and flattening of the head of the metatarsal and base of the proximal phalanx along with irregular, sclerotic bone margins and occasional loose bodies in the joint. Occasionally, the third and fourth toes can be affected. The cause is not fully understood, but it begins in adolescence as an osteochondritis – in other words, an inflammatory condition affecting both bone and cartilage. This type of finding should be reviewed by a radiologist or senior member of A&E for possible referral and to exclude a more sinister cause.

Chapter 11
Self-test quiz

This final chapter contains some images from the anatomical regions that we have covered in order to test your powers of radiographic interpretation. The answers (as we see them) are at the end of the chapter. As we have emphasized throughout this book, if you apply a systematic approach to each examination, you should be able to detect the abnormalities. Not all the images are of fractures, but all of them do have some sort of abnormality on them. The disadvantage you have is that you cannot examine the patient but are provided only with the clinical information that was on the original request form. This is, at best, sparse.

We hope that you find this a useful textbook for applying radiography as a diagnostic tool.

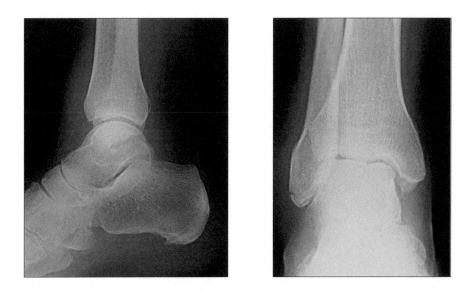

Case 1 Inversion injury. Pain and swelling. Unable to bear weight.

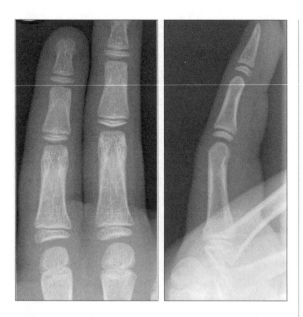

Case 2 7-year-old boy. Unclear mechanism of injury. There is bony pain and swelling of the proximal phalanx of the index finger of the right hand.

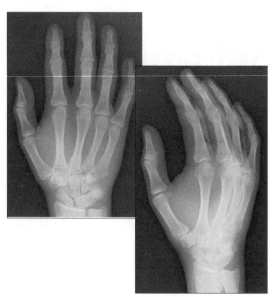

Case 3 Pain in metacarpals following heavy lifting.

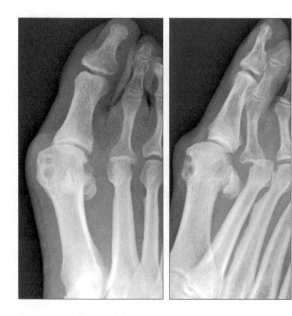

Case 4 Painful great toe. 64-year-old gentleman.

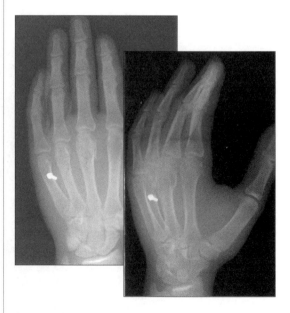

Case 5 Shot with air-gun pellet. Foreign-body localization.

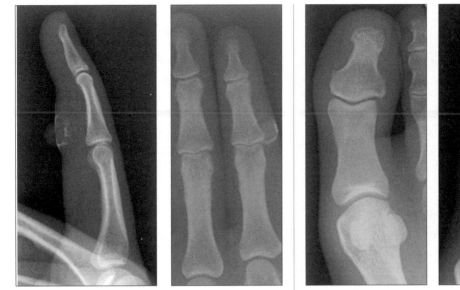

Case 6 Lump on finger – any bony involvement?

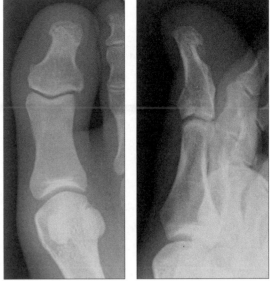

Case 7 Accidentally kicked kerbstone. Pain ++.

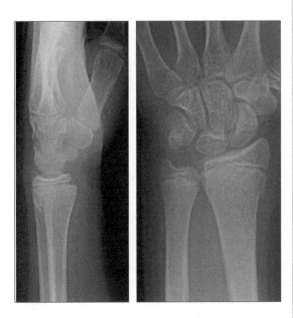

Case 8 11-year-old boy. Fell off bike. Pain in distal radius.

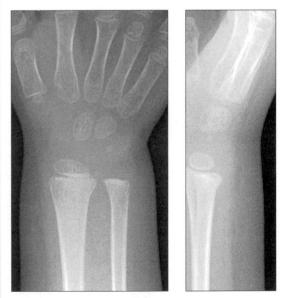

Case 9 4-year-old girl. Fell off scooter. Not using arm. (Note that only three carpal bones have ossified – can you identify them?)

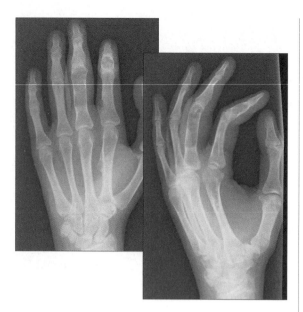

Case 10 Pain in hand following fall.

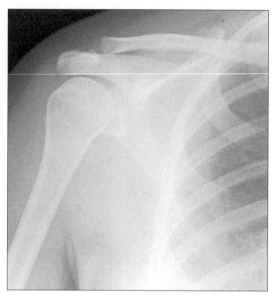

Case 11 Fell over two days ago onto outstretched arm. Pain in clavicular region.

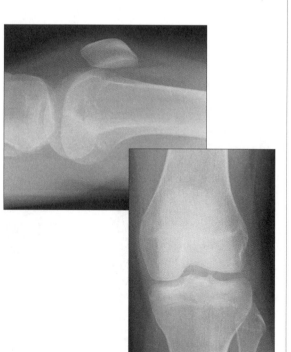

Case 12 Fell from horse. Pain in patella and proximal tibia, unable to weight-bear.

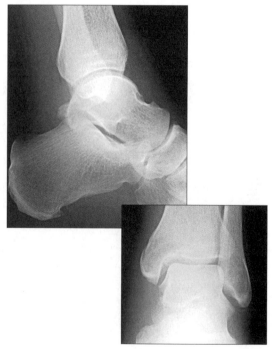

Case 13 52-year-old lady tripped and fell. Pain ++ in ankle.

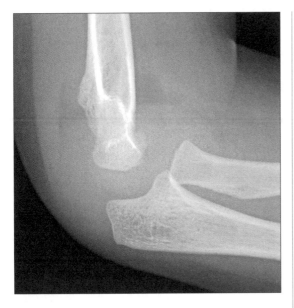

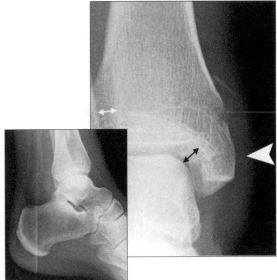
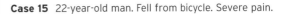

Case 14 2-year-old. Fell from swing. Not using arm. Refuses to be examined. (Only one view was achievable.)

Case 15 22-year-old man. Fell from bicycle. Severe pain.

Answers

Answer 1 There is an undisplaced fracture of the tip of the distal fibula (see detail view below. Treatment would be as for a sprain. Note that tracing the outline of the fibula on the lateral view reveals the fracture, but it is more noticeable on the AP view.

Answer 2 There is a very subtle metaphyseal fracture at the base of the proximal phalanx of the index finger. There is no break in the cortex but there is a slight buckle, best shown on the lateral view (see arrow on detail view, below).

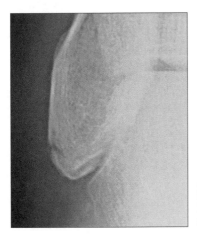

Answer 1
Fracture of tip of lateral malleolus, detail view.

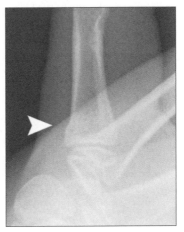

Answer 2
Metaphyseal buckle fracture.

Answer 3 This is a bit sneaky because there is no fracture; however, there is a fusion of the lunate with the triquetral – see arrow on detail view. If you traced around all the joint spaces carefully, you would have detected this. This finding is incidental and has no clinical significance.

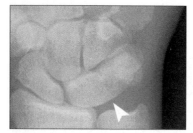

Answer 3
Developmental fusion of lunate and triquetral.

Answer 4 The metatarso-phalangeal joint of the great toe is clearly abnormal with a degree of angulation present (hallux valgus) and degenerative-type changes. However, look carefully at the joint: the appearances are not absolutely typical of osteoarthritis and another diagnosis – possibly gout – should be considered. Notice how there are what appear to be erosive lesions just next to the joint. Get an expert opinion and follow up any referral to check the outcome. This is how experience is gained.

Answer 5 The air-gun pellet is clearly visible on the films – did you also see the fractured head and neck of the third metacarpal?

Answer 6 The soft-tissue lump is clearly visible on the lateral view, as is the lack of bony involvement. The dense ring-like lesion is actually ointment. The lump is a wart that has been treated with a radiopaque cream giving the appearance shown.

Case 7 There is an intra-articular fracture at the base of the distal phalanx. It is best shown on the oblique view, detail below.

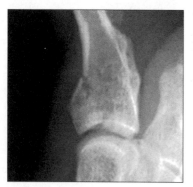

Answer 7
Detail oblique view.

Answer 8 This is not a simple distal radial fracture. The fracture line communicates with the growth plate and there is dorsal displacement of the epiphysis. This is therefore a Salter and Harris type II fracture requiring orthopaedic intervention and follow-up.

Answer 9 There is a buckle-type fracture of the distal radius, although it appears not to affect the growth plate. This is a subtle appearance but should not be missed with a careful scan of the films. The ossifying carpals are capitate, hamate and triquetral.

Answer 10 There are multiple lucent lesions seen in the index and middle fingers and the metacarpal of the index finger. You would have to get an expert radiological opinion to exclude a malignant process. In this case, the condition is multiple enchondroma, known as Ollier's disease. An enchondroma that occupies the width of a long bone will weaken the bone tissue and render it susceptible to pathological fracture.

Answer 11 There is a slight (grade I) acromio-clavicular subluxation. No other abnormality is present. Treatment is conservative.

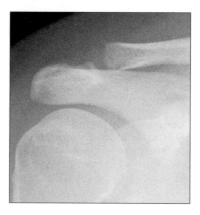

Answer 11.

Answer 12 On first inspection, no fracture is present; however, always check the lateral view of the knee. In this patient, there is a horizontal line adjacent to the patella separating blood from a fat layer – a lipohaemarthrosis. This would strongly suggest an occult (unseen) fracture and an undisplaced tibial plateau fracture should be uppermost in your mind. A CT scan may well reveal this to be the case. Follow up – get CT result.

Answer 13 There is a subtle fracture of the medial malleolus that can be seen communicating with the joint space (arrowheads on detail view, below).

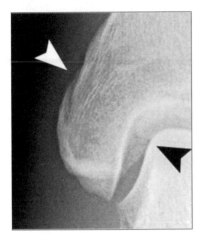

Answer 14 Unfortunately, only one view was obtainable with this little girl. However, a lateral view is diagnostic for elbow fracture. In this case, there is a large joint effusion with a prominent displacement of both fat pads, and evidence of a fracture line can be seen at the tip of the distal humerus. Appearances are of a supracondylar fracture.

Answer 15 This is a severely injured ankle, although with a quick glance this might not be fully appreciated. There is clearly a fracture of the distal fibula, which is seen on both views. Look closely at the distal tibia and at the mortice joint space. There is a fracture of the medial malleolus that communicates with the joint space (white arrowhead) and there is widening of the joint space medially and a corresponding widening of the syndesmosis (double-headed arrows – see detail view, below). This indicates an unstable joint and the patient was referred to orthopaedics for surgical fixation.

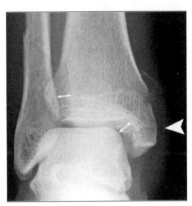

Answer 15 Fracture of the distal fibula, distal tibia and disruption of the syndesmosis.

Glossary

A&E	Accident and Emergency department
abduction	movement of a limb away from the midline (opposite of adduction)
AC joint	acromio-clavicular joint
adduction	movement of a limb towards the midline (opposite of abduction)
ALARA	as low as reasonably achievable (the intention of minimising radiation dose while at the same time giving maximum diagnostic benefit)
anatomical snuff box	depression found on the lateral aspect of the wrist formed by tendons (compression of the box is used to detect scaphoid fractures (see Chapter 6)
angulation	angle between the fragments of a fractured bone
anterior	nearer the front of the body
anterior colliculus	distal anterior tip of the fibula
anterior draw test	test used to confirm a complete tear of the anterior talo-fibular ligament (see Chapter 9)
antero-posterior (AP)	X-ray beam passes from the front of the patient to the back of the patient and then to the recording cassette
attenuation	reduction in strength of an X-ray beam due to absorption of some of the beam by an intervening material
avulsion fracture	(aka: 'flake fracture') sudden muscle/ligament/capsular contraction leading to a piece of bone being pulled off
axial compression test	(aka: 'telescoping thumb into snuff box') test used in detecting scaphoid fractures (see Chapter 6)
backslab	splint made out of plaster applied to the posterior aspect of the arm/leg
Bankhart's lesion	lesion seen in the inferior glenoid on shoulder radiographs following repeated dislocation

Barton's fracture	intra-articular fracture of the distal radius resulting in forward slip of the anterior lip of the radius
Bennett's fracture	fracture/dislocation to the base of first metacarpal (Chapter 7)
Bohler's angle	rule to help identify calcaneal fractures (see Chapter 9)
Boxer's fracture	fracture to the head/neck of fifth metacarpal (see Chapter 7)
Buckle fracture	(aka: 'torus fracture') micro fractures of the trabeculae causes cortex to buckle but remains intact (see Chapter 3)
Buddy strapping	(aka: 'neighbour strapping') splinting of finger/toe to its neighbouring digit
chondrocalcinosis	calcification of cartilage seen most often in degenerative change but also can be present with certain endocrine disorders
Colles' fracture	fracture of the distal radius within 2.5 cm of the wrist with dorsal angulation +/- impaction (associated ulnar styloid fracture may be present)
comminuted fracture	bones are splintered into two or more fragments
Compound fracture	(aka: 'open fracture') fracture where the skin has broken
CR	Computed Radiography
crescent sign	overlapping articular surfaces of glenoid cavity and humeral head (on AP view)
CRITOL rule	mnemonic system for ossification order of the paediatric elbow (see Chapter 5)
crush fracture	fracture caused by crushing injury, e.g. heavy object landing of foot – bone is crushed
c-spine	cervical spine
CT	Computed Tomography
CVA	cerebrovascular accident – generalized term for a stroke due to either infarct or haemorrhage
DIP	distal inter-phalangeal (joint)
dislocation	complete disruption of a joint where the articular surfaces are no longer in contact
displacement	bone ends have shifted in relation to each other
distal	away from the trunk or origin
dorsal	nearer the back of the body

dorsi-plantar or dorsi-palmer (DP)	refers to extremity projections; the X-ray beam passes from the top of the hand or foot to the palm or sole and then to the recording cassette
DR	Digital Radiography
enlocated	joint is located, as opposed to dislocated
Equinus plaster	plaster cast used in treating ruptured Achilles tendon – foot is in planter flexion ('equinus position')
eversion	movement of foot outwards (away from midline)
extension	opening of a joint, e.g. straightening the elbow
fabella	a sesamoid bone that exists in most people but not all
fatigue fracture	(aka: 'stress' or 'March fracture') occurs as a result of repetitive (or unaccustomed) minor stress rather than trauma
flake fracture	(aka: 'avulsion fracture') sudden muscle/ligament/capsular contraction leading to a piece of a bone being pulled off
flexion	closing of a joint, e.g. bending the elbow
fracture	disruption in the continuity of the cortex of a bone
GA	general anaesthetic
Galeazzi's fracture/dislocation	fracture shaft of the radius with dislocation of the distal radio-ulnar joint
gamekeeper's thumb	(aka: 'skier's' or 'poacher's thumb') complete rupture of the ulnar collateral ligament of first metacarpal
greenstick fracture	occurs in children – fracture is incomplete and only affects cortex on one side of the bone
Hills-Sachs' lesion	notching of the humeral head due to anterior dislocation causing impingement on the glenoid rim
impaction	one segment of bone is pushed into another
inferior	below
inversion	movement of foot 'inwards' (towards midline)
Jones' fracture	fracture to the proximal shaft of fifth metatarsal
lateral	away from the midline of the body
Lisfranc injury	fracture/dislocation of the tarso-metatarsal joint (see Chapter 10)
Maissonneuve fracture	spiral fracture to the proximal fibula with an associated fracture to the distal tibia at the ankle

Mallet finger	rupture of the extensor tendon at the distal inter-phalangeal joint (finger) leading to characteristic 'drop' of distal phalanx
March fracture	(aka: 'stress' or 'fatigue fracture') occurs as a result of repetitive (or unaccustomed) minor stress rather than trauma
McMurray's test	test used to identify damage to menisci
medial	nearer the midline of the body
MIU	Minor Injury Unit
Monteggia's fracture/dislocation	fracture of the ulna with a dislocation of the head of the radius
MRI	Magnetic Resonance Imaging
myositis ossificans	callus formation in the tissues near a joint caused by overuse or too early mobilization
NAI	non-accidental injury
neighbour strapping	(aka: 'buddy strapping') splinting of finger/toe to its neighbouring digit
oblique fracture	fracture at an angle to the length of the bone
Ollier's disease	multiple enchondromata
open fracture	(aka: 'compound fracture') fracture where the skin has broken
Os trigonum	sesamoid bone behind the talus
ossification	mineralizing process forming bone from (normally) a cartilage precursor
ossification centre	point of commencement of bone formation: primary in the shaft or main body of a bone or secondary in an epiphysis or apophysis
osteochondritis	inflammation of bone and associated cartilage
PACS	Picture Archiving and Communication Systems
pathological fracture	fracture caused by a disease process (e.g. cancer) in the bone with no or little trauma
PIP	proximal inter-phalangeal joint
plantar	sole of the foot
PMH	past medical history
poacher's thumb	(aka: 'gamekeeper's' or 'skier's thumb') complete rupture of the ulnar collateral ligament of first metacarpal
posterior	nearer the back of the body
posterior colliculus	distal posterior tip of the fibula
postero-anterior (PA)	X-ray beam passes from the back of the patient to the front of the patient and then to the recording cassette

Pott's fracture	fracture to the distal tibia (+/- fibula) and dislocation of the ankle
process	localized projection
pronation	rotating the forearm such that the palm faces down
proximal	towards the trunk or origin
radiolucent	of low density allowing X-rays to freely pass with little or no absorption
radiopaque	of high density causing significant or almost complete absorption of X-rays
RTA	road traffic accident
Salter and Harris classification	system used to classify fractures involving the growth plates (see Chapter 3, Figure 3.5)
Segond fracture	avulsion fracture of the lateral aspect of the proximal tibia adjacent to the tibial plateau
Sesamoid bone	normal accessory bone – develops within a tendon to reduce wear at sites of great stress, e.g. head of first metatarsal
Simmond's test	test used to confirm rupture of the Achilles tendon (see Chapter 9)
skier's thumb	(aka: 'gamekeeper's' or 'poacher's thumb') complete rupture of the ulnar collateral ligament of first metacarpal
Smith's fracture	fracture of distal radius with palmer displacement
spiral fracture	fracture that curves around the bone diameter
sprain	incomplete tear of a ligament, muscle or tendon as distinct from a complete tear
stress fracture	(aka: 'March' or 'fatigue fracture') occurs as a result of repetitive (or unaccustomed) minor stress rather than trauma
subluxation	minor disruption of a joint where the articular surfaces remain in some contact
superior	above – towards the head
supination	rotating the forearm such that the palm faces up
syndesmosis	non-mobile joint where the bones are united by fibrous tissues (ligament or interosseus membrane)
Terry Thomas sign	abnormally widened gap between the carpal bones caused by ligament rupture (see Chapter 6)
torus fracture	(aka: 'buckle fracture') micro fractures of the trabeculae cause cortex to buckle but remain intact (Chapter 3)

transverse fracture	fracture across the bone
tubercle	small rounded elevation
tuberosity	large rounded elevation
U-slap	plaster cast bent as a 'U' over the lateral and medial surfaces of the upper arm – used in humeral fractures
volar	on the palmer side of the hand

References

Adams N (2004) Knee injuries. Emergency Nurse 11(10): 19–27.

Allerston J, Justham D (2000) Nurse practitioners and the Ottawa ankle rules: comparison with medical staff in requesting X-rays for ankle-injured patients. Accident and Emergency Nursing 8(2): 110–15.

Bowman S, Sloane C (1999) Basic principles of diagnostic radiology. In: M Walsh, A Crumbie, S Reveley (eds) Nurse Practitioners: Clinical Skills and Professional Issues. Oxford: Butterworth-Heinemann.

Cameron A, Masterson A (2003) Reconfiguring the clinical work force. In: A Davies (ed.) The Future Health Workforce. Oxford: Palgrave Macmillan.

Cheyne N, Field-Boden Q, Wilson I et al. (1987) The radiographer and the frontline diagnosis. Radiography 53(609): 114.

Chudleigh J (2004) Nurse-requested X-rays in an A&E department. Emergency Nurse 11(9): 32–6.

Dandy DJ, Edwards DJ (2003) Essential Orthopaedics and Trauma (fourth edn.). Edinburgh: Churchill Livingstone.

Davies A (2003) A new workforce in the making? In: A Davies (ed.) The Future Health Workforce. Oxford: Palgrave Macmillan.

Dean C, Pegington J (1996) Core Anatomy for Students. Volume 1: The Limbs and Vertebral Column. London: W.B. Saunders.

Department of Health (2000) The NHS Plan: A Plan for Investment, a Plan for Reform. London: The Stationery Office.

Department of Health (2001) Reforming Emergency Care. London: The Stationery Office.

Department of Health (2003) Ten Key Roles for Allied Health Professionals. London: The Stationery Office.

Department of Health and Royal College of Nursing (2003) Freedom to Practice: Dispelling the Myths. London: The Stationery Office.

Dolan B (2000) The Nurse Practitioner: Real-world Research in A&E. London: Whurr.

Greenspan A (2000) Orthopaedic Radiology: A Practical Approach. London: Lippincott, Williams and Wilkins.

Guly HR (1996) History Taking, Examination and Record Keeping in Emergency Medicine. Oxford: Oxford University Press.

Guly HR (2002) Injuries initially misdiagnosed as sprained wrist (beware the sprained wrist). Journal of Accident and Emergency Medicine 19(1): 41–2.

Gunn C (2002) Bones and Joints: A Guide for Students. Edinburgh: Churchill Livingstone.

Helms C (1994) Fundamentals of Skeletal Radiology. London: W.B. Saunders.

Hoskote AU, Martin K, Hormbrey P et al. (2003) Fractures in infants: one in four is non-accidental. Child Abuse Review 12(6): 384–91.

Keats TE (1996) Atlas of Normal Röntgen Variants that May Simulate Disease. London: Mosby.

Knapton P (1999) Shoulder injury: a case study. Emergency Nurse 6(10): 25–8.

Lissauer R (2003) Delivering a patient-centred service. In: A Davies (ed.) The Future Health Workforce. Oxford: Palgrave Macmillan.

McNally C, Gillespie M (2004) Scaphoid factures. Emergency Nurse 12(1): 21–5.

McRae R (1999) Pocketbook of Orthopaedics and Fractures. Edinburgh: Churchill Livingstone.

Meadow R (1997) ABC of Child Abuse (third edn). London: BMJ Publishing Group.

Meek SJ, Ruffles G, Anderson G et al. (1998) Can A&E nurse practitioners interpret radiographs: a multicentre study. Journal of Accident and Emergency Medicine 15(2): 105–7.

Moore KL (1992) Clinically Orientated Anatomy (third edn.). London: Lippincott, Williams and Wilkins.

Nicholson DA, Driscoll PA (1993) ABC of Emergency Radiology: The Elbow. British Medical Journal 307(6911): 1058–62.

Nurse N, Rimmer M (2002) Musculoskeletal disorders. In: S Cross, M Rimmer (eds) Nurse Practitioner: Manual of Clinical Skills. Edinburgh: Baillière Tindall and Royal College of Nursing.

Overton-Brown P, Anthony D (1998) Towards a partnership in care: nurses' and doctors' interpretation of extremity trauma radiology. Journal of Advanced Nursing 27(5): 890–6.

Purcell D (2003) Minor Injuries: a clinical guide for nurses. Edinburgh: Churchill Livingstone.

Radiology Centennial Inc. http://www.xray.hmc.psu.edu.

Salter RB, Harris WR (1960) Injuries Involving the Epiphyseal Plate J. Bone Joint Surgery (Br) 42: 571–87.

Seaberg DC, Jackson R (1994) Clinical decision rules for knee radiographs. American Journal of Emergency Medicine 12(5): 541–3.

Seeley RR, Stephens TD, Tate P (1995) Anatomy and Physiology. London: Mosby.

Snaith B, McGuinness A, Arezina J et al. (2004) Introducing New Roles: Bridging the Gap. Synergy April: 9–11.

Steill I, Wells G, Laupacis A et al. (1995) Multicentre trial to introduce the Ottawa Ankle Rules for use of radiography in acute ankle injuries. British Medical Journal 311(6980): 594–7.

Steill IG, Greenberg GH, Wells GA et al. (1997) Derivation of a decision rule for the use of radiography in acute knee injuries. Annals of Emergency Medicine 26(4): 405–12.

Thomas A (ed.) (1995) The Invisible Light. Oxford: Blackwell Science.

Thornton A, Gyll C (1999) Children's Fractures. London: W.B. Saunders.

Touquet R, Nicholson DA, Driscoll, PA (1995) Recent advances: teaching in accident and emergency medicine: 10 commandments of accident and emergency radiology. British Medical Journal 310: 642–8.

Tye CC, Ross F, Kerry SN (1998) Emergency nurse practitioner services in major A&E departments: a United Kingdom postal survey. Journal of Accident and Emergency Medicine 15(1): 31–4.

Wardrope J, English B (1998) Musculoskeletal Problems in Emergency Medicine. Oxford: Oxford University Press.

Wilson GR, Nee PA, Watson JS (1997) Emergency Management of Hand Injuries. Oxford: Oxford University Press.

Index